man alive

Free your mind.
Reclaim your health.
Discover your true nature.

JORDAN TRAVERS

First published in Australia in 2017 by Ether Pty Ltd

CIP available from National Library of Australia

Art Direction, Graphic Design & Typesetting by Alexandra Saxby
Cover Paintograph by Victor Tondee
Nature photography by Salty Wings
Portrait photography by Andrew Kuypers
Editing by Jeff Loutit

The paper used to produce this book is a natural, recyclable product made from wood grown in sustainable plantation forests. The manufacturing processes conform to the environmental regulations in the country of origin.

Printed and bound in Australia by Moule-Print Pty Ltd, Fitzroy North.

Paperback ISBN: 978-0-6482105-0-4
E-book ISBN: 978-0-6482105-1-1

"Man. Because he sacrifices his health in order to make money. Then, he sacrifices money to recuperate his health. And then, he is so anxious about the future that he does not enjoy the present; the result being that he does not live in the present or the future; he lives as if he is never going to die, and then dies having never really lived".

- The Dalai Lama, when asked what surprised him most about humanity.

Contents

Your Ultimate Health

"Change yourself and you have done your part in changing the world".

- *Paramahansa Yogananda*

The Crash

"Jord! Are you ok?".

I couldn't respond.

I was just 16 years old - lying on the curb, gasping for a breath in the midnight air. My friend Archie was yelling for me. Everything was dark, and I was completely disorientated. My entire body was pulsing with pain, and I had no idea what had just happened.

I tried to get back on my feet, but I had no control over my lower body. The tail of a large Ford F250 truck revealed itself in the moonlight, towering above me with a crater of a dent in it. I had just crashed Archie and I into the back of a parked truck at 60km/hr.

Archie had rung the ambulance, and the owners of the truck were now holding my hand telling me my parents were on the way. My airways had been crushed by the helmet strap and every breath felt like it could be my last. I couldn't speak. I wanted to tell them I was ok despite how obviously untrue that was.

Soon my parents arrived, and then the paramedics. They administered morphine and cut my jeans to reveal a compound fracture of my left leg. The sight of the wound made my normally blood-strong mother quiver and sick. I could feel my Dad beside me, telling me "You're going to be ok". I barely believed him.

Now in the ambulance, driving down the streets I grew up in, I was beginning to lose consciousness. My mum was by my side, and the paramedic was adjusting his medical equipment. Like a dream, I was suddenly sailing high above. The vehicle's roof and the back door had vanished, and I was now looking down on myself, hand in Mum's, strapped into the medical life support. We were not driving, but rather flying through darkness with blips of purple, green and white light washing by.

The next thing I knew, I was screaming in agony; with half a dozen doctors and nurses surrounding me, trying to reorganise my crumpled lower leg, which had now swollen to the size of a soccer ball. A catheter was placed into my urethra, and I overheard someone say they may need to puncture my throat to help me get precious air into my lungs. Loud clicking sounded from the MRI machine as I had my entire body scanned for internal bleeding and haemorrhage. Bright lights shone down as I lay there, surrendering total control to my guardian angels. They were keeping me alive.

Then I woke up. It was now Tuesday. Two days had passed with me in a coma after incredibly skilled men and women put my leg back together. I was in a small room of the intensive care unit, with two nurses next to me. One of them was new. As I slowly came to, they alerted my parents who quickly came to my side. Unable to speak, I answered their questions on a whiteboard. I had a large tube down my throat connecting my lungs to the air around. Within a few hours, the nurses pulled out the tube with the help of my vomit reflex. My voice was coarse, barely audible.

Over the next week, over fifty friends, family and teachers came to visit me in my general ward bed. I remember the feminine presence of my mum and my recent ex-girlfriend there the most. Their love and support were deeply cherished as I fell in and out of a daze. I went home in a wheelchair with 116 stitches, my body gaunt, having only eaten few small hospital meals, enough to count on one hand.

The road to recovery was long and arduous. The pain was crippling, sometimes only dulled with emergency visits in the middle of the night to administer more medication. My stomach could only tolerate a few spoonfuls of cereal, and I didn't pass stool for over four weeks. It was more than three months before I could place my foot on the floor. The fresh skin on my feet made everything but polished floorboards feel like a bed of nails. I relied on my family for everything from feeding to showering. I missed out on my championship basketball season and end of school year parties. The loneliness and dependence on others made me incredibly insecure. I remember some days alone at home, yelling at the top of my lungs, at nothing in particular, tears streaming down my face.

I spiralled into a depression that lasted over two years. One sleepless night in my final year of high school, I walked to the medicine cabinet and just stared at the bottles of pharmaceuticals. I must have stood there for half an hour, estimating how many I would need to take to stop the pain I was feeling inside. A love for my brothers and parents helped me walk back to my bed that night, and to them, I am forever grateful.

Months went by, and I slowly found encouragement from stories of challenge and triumph. For inspiration, I read Lance

Armstrong's *It's Not About The Bike* and Dan Millman's *The Way of The Peaceful Warrior*. These books helped me to see that others had also gone through intense pain and come out to see a brighter world.

After my last surgery to remove the titanium metal from my leg, my Dad hired me a personal trainer. At 6"2' and an emaciated 55 kg, I thought it was a good idea too; I'm pretty sure He-Man got more girls than Skeletor. Over a 24 month period using traditional bodybuilding, we added 25 kg to my frame; I also found a new mentor in my trainer. I was starting to see the light at the end of the tunnel, just like in those inspirational books.

Once I realised I could change my health and my physical being, it was an almost overwhelming sense of empowerment. I became obsessed with the human body. Health and fitness were all I thought about. When I wasn't relearning how to walk, I was watching strongman competitions and basketball on ESPN. All through childhood, I was interested in the wider world of science and biology, but instead of being enthralled by marine life, it was now my own vessel: the human body.

I traded bodybuilding for yoga and began practising five times per week at a local studio. This practice was the single most important factor in my physical and mental rehabilitation. I had no spiritual compass for the first 19 years of my life, and it was here that I found a connection to a deeper sense of self and the profound wonderment of life.

Three years later, I was studying biomedicine and pre-medicine at the University of Notre Dame, with the dream to now become a medical doctor, just like the ones that saved my life in 2008. I wanted to specialise in trauma surgery and travel to disaster zones. I finished my degree and achieved an excellent score on my final exam.

To continue my exploration of myself and the world around me, I went backpacking in Latin America for a year, spending some time volunteering in a nursing home and on a permaculture farm. I grew more and more sure that becoming a doctor was my life's purpose. I returned older and wiser for my medical school interview, but a few months later, I learnt that my application was rejected.

After much deliberation, I relocated across the country to Melbourne to begin a new journey as a student of Osteopathy. I revisited the sciences of the human body, but this time with a greater emphasis on physical touch. Before completing the second year of my new degree, I had earned a part-time position as a trainee personal trainer at a highly regarded, boutique holistic gym with the name 5th Element Wellness (5EW).

Despite being incredibly conscious of my health over the last five years, I had always battled with it. One of my many endearing nicknames in high school was 'Phlegm Boy'. From defective digestion to mental health disorders to terrible skin conditions and debilitating allergies, I had suffered a lot by only 22 years old.

Well, I had now arrived at a wellness centre with hives from my chest up. With the stress of moving out of home, and in with my new girlfriend living on student welfare, I had dropped back to a skinny 73 kg. Starting on reception at 5:30 a.m., I was literally passing out by 10:00 a.m. My boss even sent me home early one day as I could barely string a coherent sentence together. Not the best start to becoming a beacon of health for our lovely wellness seeking clients.

I had spent tens of thousands of dollars on appointments, tests and supplements with geneticists, immunologists, and naturopaths but it often seemed that I understood more about my body than these experts did. Since my near death experience,

I had been incessantly researching holistic health from experts on podcasts, in books and blog articles; even using my bachelor's degree to help me understand peer-reviewed literature. Despite this, I struggled to gain control over my weak, tired and inflamed body.

After one blood test, I sat down with my boss, mentor and now dear friend, David O'Brien who declared that I had severe intestinal permeability and began his protocol immediately. I obliged, and within three weeks, my hives were gone. I had more energy than ever, and my chronic anxiety had nearly disappeared. I was in awe; this obviously wasn't magic, there had to be legitimate, biological factors at play. I began to learn everything that I could from my new saviour.

Dave was unlike any other practitioner I had ever met. He had no credentials and often mispronounced scientific terminology, but he was 6% body fat all year round at 40 years of age, while working 70 hour weeks. Most importantly, he was helping me reach a new level of health that no-one else could do.

One semester later, and I dropped out of university to pursue my new ambitions of becoming a holistic personal trainer. I was on a new path and loving it. With a background in medical science, I quickly learned to read blood panels and offer my expertise to those suffering like I was.

I was passing on my newly found knowledge and getting great results for my clients. Time and time again, I coached these busy men and women to look and feel many years younger in just a few weeks of changes to their lifestyle. I grew more and more confident in my expertise helping people achieve their goals, and within 1.5 yrs I had progressed to senior level coaching at the club. I reviewed blood work and wrote diet plans and exercise programs. I taught people to juggle, do handstands, lift hundreds of kilograms, and do the splits. I showed people the power of meditation and breathwork. I coached people to use that power in 60-degree saunas and 0-degree ice baths.

Most importantly, I empowered people to view their health as one of the most important things in their lives. They grew in confidence. Their smiles grew wider, and laughs became louder. This was as deeply fulfilling for me as it was for them. I watched thousands of people pass through the doors of 5EW, and use the simple steps that I will outline in this book, to have their health and ultimately their lives, drastically enhanced.

Your Time is Now

I often saw myself on a path to preventative medicine, but now, as a coach who interacts with someone multiple times per week, I truly feel like I have discovered this way of healing. I'm not talking about massaging someone's aura here; I genuinely have the ability to truly change someone's habits, to help them adopt a new lifestyle and reap the rewards, not just in health, but in their whole life. Please don't confuse this with hubris, I only speak from the results I (and the team at 5EW) have observed using this system. I really hope for you to implement the strategies in this book to see the same emphatic results.

Integrating the habits and principles of this book into your way of living may be the most profoundly productive activity you could do. According to the Australian Bureau of Statistics, approximately 88.5% of deaths in males aged 45-64 result from chronic (mostly preventable) diseases such as cancer, diabetes, circulatory, and respiratory diseases. Additionally, in Steve Biddulph's *The New Manhood*, he states, "Men, on average live for six years less than women do. They also have higher death rates in every age category, 'from womb to tomb'... Mental health, physical health, and mortality - men win the prize in every category. Just being male is the biggest risk factor of all".

With this understanding, it's clear the Australian male is in a problematic situation. The majority of us spend our lives pursuing a career and supporting a family, often at the expense of our health and happiness. From an evolutionary perspective, this makes sense: the hunters would risk their lives to venture off and find precious protein, while the gatherers stayed close to camp, minding the offspring for the next generation. If a man died on a hunt, it was worth the risk; for a woman to disappear from the tribe; a tragedy.

Along with this workaholic mentality, we see an enormous divorce rate and too many children who feel like they didn't get to spend enough time with Dad. The ripple effect can be catastrophic, with approximately 21.5% of deaths of men aged 15-44 resulting from suicide[1], over three times more likely than females[1]. Equally as unsettling is the fact that 80-90% of children with learning and behavioral disabilities are also male[2].

Something has to change. Men need to prioritise themselves; I don't mean a fancier car or new iPhone, I mean we need to tend to our body and mind to live a more vibrant and fulfilling existence. Most of the world's top CEOs prioritize their health as much as their wealth. Mark Zuckerberg, Richard Branson, Jeff Bezos, Tim Cook, Anthony Robbins. All these men are in excellent physical and mental condition, even while running billion-dollar companies.

To the female reader, I have a simple message. Thank you for having the courage to take responsibility for your health and the well-being of your family; you have immeasurable power to effect positive change on the people closest to you. The majority of the information within this book is also applicable to your unique biology; I am confident that if you use the methods and practices within, you too will achieve a heightened level of health and vitality that you never thought possible. As always, listen to your body.

Within health, the issues can be diverse. From chronic pain and mental health, to obesity and digestive issues, problems regarding health can be embarrassing, debilitating and even deadly. With my history of chronic allergies and digestive issues, I was, in fact, knocking on the door of autoimmune conditions such as rheumatoid arthritis and would be destined for a lifetime of immunosuppressants and painkillers.

Maybe your problems are not as obvious. Perhaps you suffer disrupted sleep patterns or require coffee to keep you alert throughout your day. Perhaps you feel you just have a little weight to lose around your belly. Whatever your problem, your life would be greatly enhanced if you had full control over your level of health and fitness.

Luckily, for all problems regarding health, the real solutions are near all the same and begin with prevention. In fact, I'll take a step further and instead focus on optimisation. We not only want to prevent pain, discomfort, lethargy, and obesity, we want to optimise your mind and body for living in a state of peak performance. Peak performance doesn't of course mean you'll be running on the field for your favourite AFL team next month; rather, your body, as a system will be in complete balance.

Health and fitness can be a confusing field of knowledge. Every direction you turn, someone claims to be an expert and can solve your problems (says the guy writing such a book). It doesn't matter who you are, at some point in your life, you've been given health advice by your parents, siblings, partner, friends, enemies, doctor, naturopath, physiotherapist, or Uber driver (who insists that pasta is healthy carbs).

As diverse as the background of the advice giver, is equal to the diversity of advice given. You've heard it all. Exercise more, eat less. Don't consume fat, meat, sugar, fruit, grains, alcohol. Supplements are the fountain of youth, or maybe they're deadly.

You're confused from asking the same questions. "Is coffee good or bad? Will dairy make me healthy or sick? Should I walk, run or lift weights?". You're tired of hearing what you should and shouldn't do, then following that advice, only to become healthy for a few weeks and then return to your sick self.

Thankfully, it's time you learnt how to implement simple strategies in this book to feel like you never thought you could, with simple changes that don't require Mt Everest levels of will power.

The Four Pillars of Wellness

I haven't spent an entire career as a family doctor. I don't have kids and have never been overweight. What qualifies me to write a book on health and fitness for time poor, overworked, burnt-out, out of shape, busy, professional, family men?

Results.

I have helped coach over 100 clients one-on-one towards optimal health in every area that the term general health encompasses. From eliminating back pain to boosting libido, men who follow a simple strategy can look and feel decades younger. Many of my clients are successful business owners and executives who have sacrificed their health for their career. They seek my help to reclaim their youth and vitality so that they can do more of the things they love.

The reason I am writing this book is to provide you with a method to get in shape, become healthy, improve your mental and sexual performance (and attractiveness) so that you can live your life to the absolute fullest. When I was covered in hives and falling asleep at the front desk of 5EW, I barely had any energy for my girlfriend and sure as hell couldn't have ever managed to raise a family.

I never want you to miss a day of work that you're passionate about. I never want you to lose your desire for your partner or them to lose it for you. I never want you to feel too tired to play with your kids for hours on end. You deserve to live wholly and fully, experiencing the vibrant colour of this human experience - and optimal health is the foundational layer to unlock that experience.

That's why I devised *The Four Pillars of Wellness*. These pillars are so simple it may seem too obvious. My clients who have embodied all four pillars have undoubtedly been the ones to ultimately elevate themselves above the rest. As a result of implementing these four pillars, they've been able to increase their income, deepen their relationships and be in the best shape of their lives; physically, mentally and emotionally. All because they focused on health first.

In this book, we will first explore our mind. This is the tool that we use to construct our life. If we do not have a sound mind, how can we live healthily and happily? It's just not possible, and you're fooling yourself if you think it is. Every signal that our body receives first comes from the brain. For example, we now understand the link between the brain and the gut. That feeling of butterflies in your stomach is not a coincidence. Profound biochemical changes occur in your digestive system which reflects the state of your nervous system. You will use your mind to become clear on your ideal physical and mental state. You will learn how to use sound, meditation and breathwork to tame your mind, and you will discover the forgotten power of people and purpose which may be the most important factors for our health and happiness.

Exposure to nature is the most commonly overlooked

component of a holistic journey to optimal health. In this second section, we explore the power of heat and cold therapy, the quality of the air you breathe and the material you walk on. You will learn how to optimise your sleep and detoxify your home from harmful chemicals. Becoming more attuned to your evolutionary biology has a profound impact on your sense of wellbeing. You will begin to feel clearer, look healthier and recognise how far you have separated yourself from the 300,000 or so year old creature that you are.

In the third section, you'll learn the simple methodology for eating that I have used to help one man lose more than 60 kg of pure fat and transform his relationships with his kids. There are no crash diets, quick fixes or eight week transformations in this section. All my advice in this book is given maintaining a priority for health first, physical aesthetics second. There are plenty of bodybuilding books that will help you get on stage and become so dehydrated that you're nearly dead. This is not one of those books. By the end of this section, it is my mission to help you dispel 90% of the myths circulating the nutrition world and have a clear understanding of how to eat for optimal health.

Finally, you will learn about movement. I choose not to call it exercise as I believe in a much deeper level of human movement. I believe that our society in which we believe moving for three to five hours per week and sitting, lying or standing for the remaining 163 hours is fundamentally damaging to your health. The universe of movement is so diverse (even more diverse than nutrition) it would be impossible to cover even a tiny fraction of it in this book. However, by the end of this section, you will have a simple framework in which to be confident that you can develop your human body to look and feel good naked (admit it, you were thinking it).

You have only been given one vessel to navigate this beautiful thing called life. A lot of people are counting on you to live a long health-span, that is the amount of time that you are healthy, active and able to contribute to the world. Your children's children deserve to have an active and virile grandfather, your partner hopes for you to live as long as they do, and your community wants you to be the hero of your life's story.

You have sacrificed your health for others long enough. The time for you to prioritise your body, your one universe-navigating vessel, is now. I am excited for you, dear reader, because I know how profoundly rich your life can become if you implement the strategies contained within this book. If you are ready to take a deep dive and explore your humanness, turn the page and read this book. It is my wish that you take on this knowledge to become your best self and help the ones who depend on you for so much, see you for who you really are.

mind

Chapter One

Journey Within

"Content makes poor men rich; discontentment makes rich men poor".

- Benjamin Franklin

Before we learn about my greatest tips and tricks to become a thriving human being, I want you to take a moment to contemplate the reason you're reading this book. Of course, becoming as healthy as possible has merit on its own, but in my experience, there is always a driving force behind someone's decision to become healthier. Some of the most rewarding moments as a coach have not come from teaching someone the mechanics of a squat, but by diving within a student's psychology that brought them to me in the first place.

These coaching sessions often involve finding out their major goals, like dropping body fat, reducing back pain or creating more energy, but I often try to understand why they have these goals. When a 200 kg man works into a holistic wellness centre, there is a deep, driving force that allows him to wade through dozens of judgemental eyes of fit, healthy people. This driving force is what I am interested in.

In the case of this (formerly 200 kg) client who is now my close friend, he has three young sons who he wanted to be around for. He wanted to be able to walk across the street to watch his boy play footy. He wanted to be able to dance with them at their family events. He wanted to see them grow old and have them be proud to call this man their father. I'm happy to say that in just a couple short years, he has achieved this and can now keep up with his boys all day long.

To achieve greatness in any field, you must first define what greatness looks like. You must give yourself a few moments in a quiet space to identify what it is that you want. It can be health related, or perhaps some other goal that you're working toward. It doesn't matter what your 'ideal' looks like - what is important, is that you are deeply connected to this new reality.

Being able to identify your new reality is important, but just as important, is being able to connect with your vision regularly. To connect on a daily or weekly basis with your vision - your reason *why* - is just as important as identifying this reason in the first place. Throughout your journey, you will need to find a regular time and space to craft the skill of contemplation and connect within. We're not talking about achieving enlightenment here, just a few quiet moments to reflect on why you're doing this. This sort of self imposed, albeit temporary, silence is a key to this journey.

Finding space to allow yourself to journey within is sometimes difficult. From family and work obligations to religious and cultural commitments, often we can pack our calendar so full of 'doing things' with, and for other people, that we truly forget to be with ourselves. It seems that in modern society, giving ourselves space and silence are the most difficult gifts we can offer. There's always someone's special event or a last-minute project to complete. The phone always beeps with an 'urgent' email. But the magic of silence is something that we cannot deprive ourselves of if we want to live a happy and fulfilling life.

Where there is silence, there can be listening, and we begin to understand our inner self with much more clarity. We can start to hear our intuition, our deepest needs and desires and whether or not we are on the right path to fulfilment. This is when true happiness occurs.

So how are you to find this silence? Put simply, you must create it. There are a few ways, which I've found to be useful that allow my inner voice to come forward. You can take a full day out by yourself and hike in nature, with no technology and no one else around or you can take just one or two hours and book a massage or sensory deprivation tank.

These tanks are filled with 500 kg of magnesium salts in water that is heated to your body temperature. You close the lid to lay in complete darkness, with every one of your senses able to 'turn off' and relax. Here you let yourself float into stillness and allow yourself just to *be*. With reduced cerebral activity, your mind and body can repair very quickly. If that sounds somewhat claustrophobic by the way, try and think of it as the exact opposite: of lying in infinite space. One of my clients recently described a feeling of dissolving into oneness with everything. Because he could not see, hear, feel anything, he said that he no longer identified with himself and for a few moments he became no time, no space and no one. I let him know that he achieved the state that yogis strive to reach for decades. Funnily enough, he didn't seem too phased.

Another option, which requires more flexibility, is to go on retreat. Whether it is a 10 day silent meditation retreat or simply a few days in Bali doing yoga twice per day and eating healthy food, I have found these experiences to be incredibly invaluable for me to reach a state of peace and clarity within myself. This presence allows me to recalculate my vision and direction I have for myself and I go back home with more coherence and focus on growing.

Not all means of contemplation require you to venture to

faraway lands, don a hemp cape, or even leave your home. A regular practice of journaling has a profoundly calming effect on your nervous system. I have often said that I don't have enough time to journal, but when I do, I feel much more connected to myself and my path. The worries of daily life seem insignificant after a 10-20 minute period of journaling. By talking to myself with a pen to paper, I suddenly have new insights into problems and gain a different perspective on life. You'll be amazed at what seeing your underlying thoughts written on paper can do in terms of holding those issues to an objective light.

I was most consistent with journaling while travelling through Latin America. To give you an idea into what this process looks like, here's an unedited journal entry from 17 June 2013 when I was living on a yoga-permaculture farm in Costa Rica.

"Talking to Mary today about trusting the flow of life was very important. I feel like I am already in Med School and have faith I will be accepted – or perhaps I'll be safely redirected to another path.

I have realised that I will leave the yoga teaching to the best for the current moment. Treat yoga as you feel it. It is not your entire life. Don't force it. Be natural in the practice and enjoy the path along. No need to study the dharmas, dogmas, etc. Feel the movement, breath and energy as they arise. We're not chasing the yogic dragon here. Learn the lessons: loving kindness, compassion, stillness, tranquillity, non-judgement, equanimity, ego-transcendence, humility. Let those flow through the river of your entire being.

It is important to have integrity by walking the talk and fulfilling what is asked of you. Always have gratitude for the people that surround you for they provide you with love, laughter and life lessons. Be honest in every sense.

I get to see my beloved family in 3 weeks. Get excited you big f*ck! Boom!

On the road for six months today. Congratulations Jordy-boy. You have come a very long way. Keep on playing and dance the dance of life.

Namaste Motherf*cker".

I found this self-talk to be incredibly therapeutic. It's a form of self-imposed psychoanalysis that brings up your subconscious thoughts and understandings. Letting go of perfect grammar or the need to make sense allows the free-flow of consciousness to give direct access to rewrite your neurochemistry. Sometimes, I moved from a state of depression and confusion to total gratitude in a few short minutes with this method of scribbling to the self.

The Five Minute Journal is a tool that some of my clients and I have used to spend a little time reconnecting with ourselves. In it, you write down what you want to achieve in the day, what you are grateful for and how you want to be. You also have the option at the end of the day to review your day and think of ways to make it better. This tool has positively impacted the lives of some of my clients, where they now seek things to be grateful for throughout the day, so that they have something to write in their journal. They now notice the song of birds in the trees or the laughter of a baby in the checkout. It's the small things that count; those little moments of observation and wonder will quickly make that presentation tomorrow seem a bit less stressful.

All of these introspective practices allow you to clear the mental debris from your daily life. Whether it be hiking alone in nature or sitting down in your living room with a pad and pen, I find that these practices significantly improve the quality of my life and act as a mental reboot. It feels like I am emptying out the trash of my mind to make space for new and interesting thoughts and ideas to come forward. The investment of time

...to rebooting my mind pays incalculable dividends for the future.

Studies have shown that a regular practice of journaling, particularly about the things we are grateful for, is very effective at reducing our levels of stress and enhancing our happiness[3]. For most people in today's society, this is probably the one thing that we are all striving for. Less stress, more happiness. When we are in this state of peace and clarity, we can make better decisions in business, in our relationships and within ourselves to ultimately live a richer, more fulfilling life.

So your first task is this: I want you to spend a maximum of 10 minutes each day writing in a journal for the next seven days.

First you must complete the following:

1. Define your ideal state of health.
2. Write down *how* you want to look and feel within your body.
3. Detail what your daily life looks like.
4. Get clear on your *why* of reading this book.
5. Write down *who* you are doing this for.
6. Write the challenges you want to overcome and the feelings that will result of these achievements.
   Be specific. Be detailed.

Once you've done that, just allow anything else to come. I want you to write terribly, with improper grammar and spelling and just to write as many shitty words as you can. The faster you write, the better. Try not to stop. Preferably use a pen and paper, but if you must, you can use a computer. Typing on a tablet or smartphone doesn't allow you to fully let go or get in the zone. This is about tapping into your subconscious and revealing your true self. Nobody is watching.

Journeying within to get clear on your ideal reality and your reason *why* is your first task for this book. If you do this with full intent, you will be much more likely to take the steps I outline in the following chapters. If you feel inclined, put down the book now, place a 10-minute timer beside you and get scribbling. Allow the mental download to occur. You will be healthier for it.

Chapter Two

Don't Worry, Be Happy

"The desire to know your own soul will end all other desires".

- *Rumi*

Now that you've made space for contemplation and begun the journey within, it's time to take the next step and learn about the way to prevent the single biggest killer of human beings. This phenomenon is so strong that it's likely that every chronic disease known stems from this one factor. The unsettling thing about this is that we deliberately choose to expose ourselves to this every single day. This phenomenon is known as stress.

When we are stressed, we cause a cascade of hormones that break down the body including our muscle mass and the structure of our brain. A hormone that you will see mentioned a lot in this book is called cortisol. Before working at 5EW, despite studying biomedical science, pre-medicine and osteopathic medicine, I wasn't that well aware of the effects of cortisol. In fact, I had probably only heard it mentioned a handful of times throughout my five and a half years of university education.

Thankfully I was able to learn on the battlefield about the effects of chronic cortisol elevation. Every one of my clients, and even my colleagues and myself were consistently overexposing ourselves to this hormone. From immune suppression to gut dysfunction there aren't many functions of the body that aren't affected by cortisol, either directly or indirectly. However, this hormone is not evil. It is simply the chronic elevation of this hormone in our blood that is detrimental to our health.

Cortisol exists to help us run or fight against danger; y'know, the 'oh my god there is sabertooth tiger chasing me caveman type deal'. The trouble is, we don't have to worry about that sort of loincloth-filling fear anymore, but our bodies have found a way to simulate that thanks to modern society. Our bodies now think we are running or fighting against danger all day, every day for the entire year.

Most people I meet tell me that they're not stressed, so I like to offer up a different word. Stimulated. We humans are more stimulated in our modern lives than ever. When a mobile phone pings in your pocket, that's stimulation. When a plane flies overhead - stimulation. Renowned strength coach, Charles Poliquin has suggested that due to technology and our modern responsibilities, we are approximately 100 times more stimulated than our great grandparents. This stimulation doesn't come without consequences.

Humans are unique in that we can think of a situation, and it causes the same effect within our body. When you imagine losing money in a deal that hasn't happened yet, or you visualise a fight with your partner that only exists within your mind, you create a fear response in your brain. This in turn sets off a rainbow of beautiful stress hormones that say 'stop everything and *run*'. But you can't, because you're in your car, and jumping into oncoming traffic would be stupid, so you ruminate some more.

Negative rumination increases cortisol and corticotropin-releasing hormone that tells your body to break down proteins, spike blood sugar levels, destroy neurons in your brain, open holes in your intestinal wall and many other unhappy functions.

The beautiful thing about all this is that we can do something about it. That something is called meditation.

Meditation is the act of taming the mind to become aware of, and completely immersed in the present moment. The ideal state is that our internal thoughts reflect the immediate external world of what is happening around us. Notice how I mentioned that this is the ideal state. I say this because (and I'm sure you've heard this before), many people say that they can't meditate because they *think too much*. This is the same as someone saying they can't do yoga because they're too inflexible or that they can't change their diet and move more because they're too overweight. It's insane to use the reason for an action as the excuse not to do it.

The benefits of meditation are almost endless. Over 100 genes can change within minutes of meditation[4]. These genes are associated with reduced levels of inflammation and risk of chronic disease. As far as epigenetic (gene-altering) lifestyle habits go, meditation is one of the top activities you can do to rewrite your genes for a healthier future.

Of course, there are many different types of meditation. From mindfulness to meta, various methods of meditation are used for different outcomes. The most common practice, which is one that I recommend for beginners, is mindfulness. It involves focusing on the sensations of the surrounding environment. The focus could be the birds singing, the rise and fall of your abdomen while breathing, or a truck siren in reverse. It doesn't always have to be profound and spiritual. When you realise you are thinking about something else, which you inevitably will, you go back to focusing on the birds. And when you realise you are thinking again, you go back to focusing on the birds. Catch yourself, bring yourself back. Rinse and repeat, and you're meditating.

Numerous guided meditations are flooding the internet. Sam Harris, Dan Harris, Tara Brach, *Headspace*, and *Calm* all begin with simple mindfulness techniques to clear away the mental chatter and connect you deeper to yourself. If you are seeking more expansive and enlightening experiences, I recommend the longer meditations from Dr Joe Dispenza, although these are not for beginners.

If you prefer to go alone, a simple method is just to sit and try not to move. Become acutely aware of everything that you feel, from the pressure of your legs from your seat to the beating of your own heart. Spending 10 minutes in the morning bringing your awareness inward can help you achieve peace and clarity before you get on with your day. Pairing this technique with breathwork or music can have incredibly powerful effects on your physical and mental state.

I'll confess that I don't practice meditation every day. I used to feel guilty about this until I heard Arnold Schwarzenegger on *The Tim Ferriss Show* talk about his experience with Transcendental Meditation. He practised for two years in his early adult life and had found the benefits have stayed with him for decades later. I believe to some degree, the same has happened to me. With four years of a dedicated yoga practice, I learnt how to connect to myself, and my breath. I learnt how to change my state of being to feel intense surges of gratitude, peace and contentment. I discovered that I was not who I thought I was and to have faith in something greater than myself. It often takes reminding, but by letting go and trusting that life already is perfect as it is, I feel infinitely more content with my existence.

So now and then when I feel overwhelmed with life's daily responsibilities, I will set aside some time to connect back in. It's not that I don't think meditation is necessary for me anymore. It is simply not high enough on my list of priorities until I feel like I need it. The key concept here is that I put in the work for

a few years. I journeyed into a world of unknown and l
fear time and time again. It is fear that ultimately creates these
stress responses which cause damage to our body.

On the other side of fear is gratitude. Gratitude is a state
of being in which you relinquish all attachments and are
immensely content with your current reality. It is a skill that
can, and should, be nurtured. When you become grateful for
what is, you release a cascade of endorphins that surge through
your body. These happy hormones are profoundly healing and
also very pleasurable.

The perfect gratitude meditation:

1. Take a moment to sit up straight with your eyes closed.
2. Focus your attention on the area in the middle of your chest.
3. Take five slow deep breaths into that space.
4. Now, as you inhale, visualise your breath coming down the front of your body down to your pelvis.
5. As you exhale, imagine the breath leaving the base of your spine, up the back of your body and through the tip of your head.
6. After about ten cycles, bring to mind someone who you genuinely love. Someone who has helped you become who you are today.
7. Visualise them.
8. Keep breathing slow and deep.
9. See them smiling and happy.
10. Every exhale, silently say to them "I love you. Thank you".
11. When you are ready, take a deep breath inwards, and hold it at the top for a few moments.
12. Exhale to release.
13. When you are ready, open your eyes.

This is a form of loving kindness meditation and has been shown
to create the happiest people on the planet, determined by

measuring brain waves of a Tibetan Buddhist Monk, Matthieu Ricard. A neuroscientist at the University of Wisconsin, Richard Davidson conducted a study on Ricard and showed that when meditating on compassion, his brain produces a higher level of gamma waves – those linked to consciousness, attention, learning, and memory. The neurochemistry he created allows him an abnormally large capacity for happiness and a reduced propensity towards negative emotions[5].

Don't worry if you aren't able to notice any changes immediately. As I mentioned before, this is a skill that can be crafted; you probably sucked at your first day at work too. You will find different meditations work better for you. This is a personal journey, and I'm only here to encourage you to get the journey started.

If you're someone who is chronically stimulated due to your busy life, I highly urge you to value yourself enough to learn this powerful skill. Meditation has changed the lives of and help create the world's top performers. For some people, as was the case with myself, it has cured mental health issues, and for others, even greater transformations have occurred.

So choose a time of the day where you can be alone with your thoughts for just a few minutes. This time may be directly before or after your journaling time, or it may be at the end of a yoga class. To hone this skill, you will create countless positive changes to not just your physical health, but to your decision-making skills and overall well-being. Just sit there, breathe and watch what arises. See your thoughts as clouds that glide across the horizon. They come, and they go. This is meditation.

Chapter Three

Breath of Life

"I do not fear death. I fear not to live fully".

- Wim 'The Iceman' Hof

I have had the privilege of learning from some remarkable masters of their craft, and this is especially true in the world of breathwork. For many of you, breathing exercises may be entirely foreign, and they might even seem a little too 'new age' for something that you wish to explore. That's ok, I was there once too. Luckily I was younger and had fewer layers to peel back to reveal the truth. We overlook breathing, perhaps logically, because it's innate; we don't really consciously control it, because we don't have to. But breathing is a primal skill that if you become proficient in, can be utterly life changing.

I want to take you to a particular moment in my life when I caught a glimpse of its power. I was on retreat on The Great Ocean Road, Victoria, Australia, in the middle of winter, with a special man named Wim Hof. Wim, nearly 60 years old, has claimed 26 world records in unrelated feats of human performance. His resume is crazy, being the first man to:

1. Climb 7,500m up Mt. Everest in just his shorts.
2. Run a marathon in the Namib desert without water.
3. Hang for the longest time from one finger, 500m above the earth, between two hot air balloons for a total of 29 seconds.

At an early age, Wim became fascinated with the cold and began cutting holes into iced lakes to jump in and feel the immense effect it had on his body. The icy water made him feel fully alive, forcing him to breathe intensely as if to be clutching onto life. If you've ever had a cold shower, and thought that was a shock, Wim would like a word with you. In the decades to come, Wim would continue to experiment with cold exposure and breath techniques and go on to inspire those interested in 'human optimisation' the world over.

On the fifth day of the retreat, after a beautiful day spent swimming at a nearby dam in the middle of a Victorian winter, Wim signalled everybody into the yoga hall for an unplanned breath session. He suggested we go slowly. "Fully in. Let go". His mantra repeated. The lights turned off. "Fully in. Let go".

Over the next 90 minutes, sixty people bunched together, shoulder to shoulder, breathed deeper, fuller, and longer than we had ever done in our entire lives. The power of this technique came to the surface. After one hour, my hands, arms and face, started to contort with the unique gaseous exchange and pH change occurring in my body.

Upon retention and squeezing my breath into my head, I would revisit childhood memories for what seemed like days, only to come back a few seconds later and realise I was in a room full of adventurous people. I would go again and again until the pressure in my body became too much, and so I sat up and watched in awe.

I was at genuine peace and in absolute gratitude for the world and the people in my life. I believe that this ultimately the goal of any spiritual endeavour: to make you a better person. To allow you to live a fuller life and love the world around you. It is done to make you happy, and this is the role of breathwork.

Wim is currently examining his techniques with multiple universities, including Hanover and Stanford. Not because he wants to see if there is proof - he already knows - but to prove to the current scientific community that we do not yet fully understand the frontiers of human nature. There is much more of our physiology that we are not able to access with our current toolkit. This method will show you how.

Some research has shown considerable physiological effects of the Wim Hof Method (WHM). There is a robust increase of the excitatory neurotransmitter, epinephrine, as well as an increase in oxygen saturation of the tissues from 16% to 22%[6]. By decreasing carbon dioxide levels, we can also raise the blood pH from 7.4 to approximately 7.8[6]. This state of voluntary sympathetic nervous system activation, blood alkalinity, and oxygen saturation has profound effects[6]:

1. Increased endurance.
2. Increased pain and cold tolerance.
3. Improved cardiovascular conditioning.
4. Increased white blood cell count.
5. Suppression of inflammatory cytokines.
6. Feelings of love, connection and happiness.

I have personally experienced the immune regulating effects of the WHM. During a period of peak work stress, eczema on my face reappeared. I was in Mullumbimby, New South Wales, Australia, at a coaches' retreat, when we practised the method. After just one round of 40 breaths and the rash on my face was gone. It had completely disappeared. It's incredible to imagine how many tubes of eczema cream or packets of anti-histamine tablets are used every day when we could simply use the power of our own breath to regulate our immune system.

To learn the life-changing magic of The Wim Hof Method, you can complete the 10-week online course or find a certified instructor near you via the WHM website.

I have also been able to spend time in India, learning in the Himalayas from a master by the name of Yogrishi Vishvketu, creator of Akhanda Yoga. I was fortunate enough to spend five weeks living in his ashram, learning and practising yogic postures, breathwork and mind control every day.

Pranayama is a Sanskrit word we use for breathwork that means 'life-force without restraint'. Yogis believe that breath is life, and the way in which we use our breath can dictate the way we navigate through this world. If it is short and fast, our mind is quick and agitated; if it is deep and slow, the mind is calm and content.

There are a few simple explanations for this. Firstly, when our diaphragm contracts and pushes our abdominal organs down and out, this triggers our major parasympathetic nerve, the vagus nerve. The parasympathetic nervous system (PNS) governs our rest and digest facilities, making us calm and relaxed. Secondly, when we breathe deep, we deliver more oxygen to the tissues throughout the body and in particular, the brain. When the brain has oxygen, we are happy. When it doesn't have oxygen, not so much.

Another way Yogis increase oxygen delivery is, counterintuitively, by holding the breath. The Bohr effect says that when carbon dioxide levels rise in the blood, there is a faster delivery of oxygen from the blood into the surrounding tissues. To capitalise on this, we breathe a lot for a short period (one to five minutes), then hold the breath. After increasing oxygen levels, we increase carbon dioxide and diffuse more oxygen from the bloodstream into the tissues.

To trigger the PNS, we hold the breath out; to trigger the sympathetic nervous system, we hold the breath in. The area in our brain that regulates our emotion, the Limbic System, is also the centre for autonomic breath control. This relationship is why we may experience a release of emotions during intense sessions of pranayama breathwork.

By drawing out the exhalation, we also feel a deeper sense of relaxation via the PNS. Another way of drawing out the exhalation is by humming. Humming is used to soften the mind and muscles through the release of nitric oxide. We breathe in deeply and hum like a happy honey bee for as long as we comfortably can. Combine this with an infrared sauna or a sensory deprivation tank and watch yourself launch into outer space from the third person.

Through breathing techniques, we can strengthen the breathing muscles, namely the diaphragm and intercostal muscles, which can allow us to breathe deeper and easier at rest. If you have ever felt short of breath or tight in the chest due to stress or anxiety, you have lost full control over your respiratory muscles. You have lost control of the most basic and urgent system for your survival.

Babies breathe through their nose down deep into their diaphragm. Their belly expands on the inhale and falls on each exhale. The only exception is when they are sick, or when they are crying. They also have perfect squatting form, but that's for another chapter.

It is your job to now place a heightened level of awareness on how you breathe throughout the day. Is your breath short, choppy and through your mouth? Do you breathe with your accessory muscles into your chest? You may be spending too much time living in your sympathetic nervous system, your 'flight and fight' nervous system and your breathing patterns become arrhythmic and volatile.

Instead it's much healthier to breathe *less*. Counterintuitively, breathing less is actually an effective method to calm your nervous system.

Try five minutes of Box Breathing and see how you feel. Sit up straight and repeat the following steps:

1. Inhale for a count of four.
2. Hold the breath for a count of four.
3. Exhale for a count of four.
4. Retain for a count of four.

If you feel out of breathe or panicky, your tolerance to carbon dioxide (CO_2) is very poor, which indicates you're not breathing properly throughout the day due to stress or some breathing dysfunction. The more frequently we breathe during the day, the less CO_2 we have in our blood, which, according to the Bohr effect, is actually an undesirable situation. A higher tolerance to CO_2, and therefore the less you need to breathe, equates to higher levels of health and fitness[7]. In my own experience, a person with a longer out-breath retention has a healthier body and calmer mind than someone who can only hold their breath out for a few seconds. A simple test of your CO_2 tolerance comes from Dr Konstantin Buteyko:

1. Sit up straight with a stopwatch in hand.
2. Take 2 normal breaths.
3. After exhaling the second time, hold your breath out until you feel a definite desire to breathe.

According to Dr Buteyko the amount of time you hold your breath out can indicate the following[5]:

40 to 60 seconds:
Indicates a normal, healthy breathing pattern and excellent physical endurance.

20 to 40 seconds:
Mild breathing impairment, moderate tolerance to physical exercise and potential for health problems in the future (most people fall into this category).

10 to 20 seconds:
Significant breathing impairment and poor tolerance to physical exercise; nasal breath training and lifestyle modifications are recommended.

Less than 10 seconds:
Serious breathing impairment, very poor exercise tolerance and chronic health problems.

Where do you fall on this spectrum? Interestingly, this test can be used to determine how much stress you have subjected your body to over the last few days. By practicing to slow down your breathing and therefore breathe less, you are training your nervous system to remain calm in the face of stress.

I hope it's clear to you that being aware of your breath is to be aware of your life. It's incredibly beneficial to begin your day with a practice of breathwork. Whether it's The WHM, Box Breathing or another practice, the people I know who have consistently performed 10 minutes of focused breathing exercises every morning, are those who dramatically alter their physical and mental health.

These same people find themselves living each day with intent, and grow to become very healthy and conscious human beings. You deserve to wake up and experience this level of awareness. The people in your life are counting on you. All it takes is 5-10 minutes each morning to unlock your true potential.

Chapter Four

The Secret to Longevity

"Life's most persistent and urgent question is, 'What are you doing for others?'".

- *Martin Luther King Jr.*

Since homo sapiens grew conscious enough to realise our impending demise, we have attempted to quench our thirst for immortality; whether it be from the fountain of youth in the fifth century BCE, or the chalice of cosmetic surgery today. Science has in fact found many correlations of longevity, from grip strength to the ease of getting up and down on the floor, but none more evident than a cluster of atoms called telomeres.

Since Francis and Crick made revolutionary discoveries regarding DNA, the scientific understanding of longevity has continued to expand at a rapid pace. We have mapped the entire human genome. We have modified genetic material inside a human embryo. We have even identified the exact genetic material that can determine the length of the rest of our lives. But still, most of us die at 80 years old. Sick, weak, and wondering what we could have done differently.

In their book, *The Telomere Effect: A Revolutionary Approach to Living Younger, Healthier, Longer*, Nobel Prize Winners Dr Elizabeth Blackburn and Dr Elissa Epel detail how to increase not just your lifespan, but your healthspan (being the number of years that you remain healthy and active). These scientists discovered that telomeres are repetitive sequences of DNA at the end of your chromosomes that protect it from damage, much like the cap protects a shoelace from fraying.

When telomeres get shorter over time, you're moving closer to not being around anymore. We understand the damage that smoking, alcohol, stress, and lack of sleep has on telomeres. We also know the support that healthy food, exercise, and meditation gives to our telomeres. We've even discovered telomerase, an enzyme that not only prevents the shortening of telomeres but can lengthen it. Science doesn't know if this translates into the reversal of the ageing process just yet, but that doesn't stop supplement companies selling their magic herbs to you at a premium.

What we do know however, is that stress reduction is one of the most powerful supportive mechanisms to our telomeres. Chronic cortisol elevation is a tremendous way to age our bodies, from the bones in our legs to the skin on our face; there isn't a cell in our body that's not damaged by chronic stress. Here lies the secret to longevity.

In his TED Talk, *How to live to be 100+*, Dan Buettner travelled around the world to the six 'Blue Zones'; areas with a high percentage of centenarians. Among them, Okinawa Japan, Nosara Costa Rica, Ikaria Greece, and Sardinia Italy. He explained there were similarities in their diet, such as a diet of no commercially processed foods but instead locally made and grown vegetables, wine, cheese and meat. Some groups ate lots of grains while others ate small amounts. Some groups ate animal protein, and others ate minimally. What Buettner also noticed was that all inhabitants of 'Blue Zones' had a very close group of people to call their community.

These communities were so marked that they knew everything

about one another. For example, in the highlands of Okinawa, Japan, everybody belongs to a *Moai*: a group that meets weekly to discuss all things physical, spiritual, sexual, mental, financial and so on. These groups continue from early childhood until their final days passed a century. Imagine the bonds you would form with someone over an 80-90 year period of life; it certainly beats the hundreds of superficial relationships we collect on Facebook.

In late 2016, three close male friends and I came together to start our *Moai*, which we later named *Man Night*; a dinner and chat amongst mates every Thursday night. Sometimes these conversations lasted until midnight and would have kept going had we not needed to go to work the next day. I have found incredible healing occurs as we discuss masculinity, relationships, vulnerability, and other complex social struggles. We celebrate each other's wins and support one another during times of loss. The whole experience brings a profound perspective that I am not in this life alone. I have people that count on me for support, and I rely on them. This is a true tribe.

Growing up in Australia, friendships were usually about getting as drunk as possible, and maybe with enough biochemical assistance, you'd share something that's on your mind. Only when your inhibitions have been utterly annihilated, do you confide with a close friend. If this sounds familiar, I encourage you to be brave and start one of your own Man Nights. Find a group of men who are willing to be vulnerable and share what's on their mind. Eat some food and then sit down to ask each other, "How's life at the moment?". With repetition, you'll be amazed what comes up.

I remember when I first began yoga with a small group i I formed close relationships with the teachers very qu' was hooked on the peaceful, connected feeling I had class. This group called Yogaworx, started off small. S it was the teacher Wendy, myself and just one other person on a weeknight. But over time, I watched the community grow to bring together sixty people on a Sunday morning. I knew most people by name, and we would hang out after class. I continued with this group for four years before moving to Melbourne. I wonder, had the community not been such a strong part of my healing process, would I have stayed so long?

Another aspect of the Okinawan way is a concept called *Ikigai*. This translates to 'reason for being', or more simply 'reason to get up in the morning'. The process of identifying your *Ikigai* often requires a deep search into the self. For one elderly lady, her reason for being was her great, great, great, granddaughter. This super grandma was asked what does it feel like when you hold her in your arms and she responded: "It feels like leaping into heaven". Your *Ikigai* is much more powerful than a goal. It defines who you are. It can be as simple as being an incredible father or as grandiose as building a fortune 500 company.

Buettner came to the surprising realisation that 'Blue Zone' communities do not have a formalised exercise regime. Instead, they organise their day around physical activities. He showed picture after picture of hundred plus-year-old men tinkering with fences and hammering stones. These men weren't just alive at 100 years old; they were strong. They knew it too.

Dr Mario Martinez has also conducted extensive research into the beliefs of centenarians and found that there is what he calls 'inclusive arrogance'. One particular hundred-year-old man interrupted Mario during an interview to point out a group of women and said "Did you see that? They were looking at me. They thought I was beautiful. They saw that I am because they are!". This old man's confidence was amusing, cheeky, and infectious. Perhaps a belief that you are young, healthy, active and beautiful may be one of the most significant contributors to a long, healthy, active and beautiful life.

Another belief that these centenarians held, or rather did not hold, was the notion of retirement. The idea that to cease the use of your mind and body to contribute to society was incomprehensible. Most happy, older men that I know, who have had successful careers are also quietly afraid of retirement, fearing that they might become bored, or worse, lose their financial nest egg. Centenarians understand that their work is as much a part of their life as their family.

This understanding places even more importance on doing what you love for work. Why live 40 years doing something you don't enjoy to spend the last 20 years doing something you do. Don't forget that those last 20 years you won't want to go jet skiing in The Bahamas due to the fear of breaking your now brittle bones. Life is now, not post-65.

What if you could live a long, healthy life of fulfilling work, with people you love and who love you too? What if you had a reason to wake up each morning and enjoyed your labour, not just it fruits? What if you lived to be over 100 and could hold your great, great, great grandson in your arms? Wouldn't that be a life well lived?

Forget about bio-hacks and understand that the length of time that you live long and healthy is determined by a deeper sense of belonging. It is determined by the strength of your tribe and the connection to your life purpose. Victor Frankl wrote a compelling book on the survival of men in Nazi camps titled, *Man's Search For Meaning* and explained that a man's purpose for survival is his only means of survival. To also quote Friedrich Nietzsche, "He who has a *why* to live for can bear almost any *how*".

The secret to longevity does not lie in some magic pill, potion or exercise equipment. It is a connection to the deeper layers of being here on the planet. Your health and longevity is dependent upon the meaning you give it. It is also dependent upon the close and meaningful relationships you have.

Let's take this time out now to write down the members of your ideal *Moai*. Contact them and tell them you want to connect and start a Man Night. I also want you to spend some time to define your *Ikigai*. Inquire deep within yourself and ask, "What is my reason to wake up in the morning?".

Part One: Mind - Summary

Experiment with journaling. Spend 10 minutes now on these questions.

1. What is your ideal state of health & fitness?
2. Why do you want to achieve this? Who will benefit?
3. What will happen if you don't achieve your ideal state? Who else will suffer?
4. What will your life be like if you achieve your ideal state?
5. If you haven't done this yet, put down the book and do it now.

Spend a few minutes each day by yourself in meditation.

6. Set a timer for 3-5 minutes.
7. Use guided meditations or apps.

Learn the power of breathing techniques.

8. Practice Box Breathing.
9. Learn the Wim Hof Method.

Surround yourself with loving people.

10. Your community is the most important factor for a happy, healthy life.

Define your *Ikigai*: Your 'reason for being'.

11. A clear and compelling purpose for life gives us immense fulfilment and well-being.

nature

Chapter Five

Start with Your Home

"Thousands of tired, nerve-shaken, over-civilised people are beginning to realise that going to the mountain is going home; that wilderness is necessity; and that mountain parks and reservations are... fountains of life".

- John Muir

Before we explore the many ways you can return to nature and attain its full benefits, we need first to investigate where you live. Instead of talking about how to bring you to the nature, it makes sense to identify how to remove as much pollution from our immediate environments as possible.

Once our sanctuary, our homes have become one of the most toxic places to lay rest. According to the Environmental Protection Agency (EPA) of the United States, levels of air pollutants inside your home may be two to five times higher than the pollution levels outside your home. Occasionally indoor air pollutant levels in studies have even reached up to 100 times greater than outdoor pollutant levels[8].

Griffith University suggests there are over 100,000 synthetic chemicals available on the household market with over 1,500 new chemicals being produced annually. Over half of these chemicals have never been tested for toxicity on the human body[9]. Tens of thousands of these chemicals can be carcinogenic, hormone disrupting, synthetic compounds used to make ourselves and our homes 'clean and beautiful'.

Grooming Yourself Healthy

Let's start with the products you directly come into contact with. Toiletries and beauty products are some of the worst culprits for poisoning your body. These everyday staples contain synthetic chemicals that can cause allergies, hair loss, skin conditions, cognitive decline, digestive issues, thyroid dysfunction, and even cancer. And if potential death wasn't quite enough to get your attention, these chemicals can also destroy your sex hormones and fertility, leading to no more adult cuddles. Over the last five decades, according to some studies, levels of testosterone and sperm count in 42,935 Western men have dropped as much as 60% between the years 1973-2011[10]. My grandfather was twice the man that I am today. Not just because he didn't wear shoes until he was 18, but also due to the oestrogenic (oestrogen creating) compounds found in my cologne.

Without a degree in organic biochemistry, it's impossible to make sense of the labels on the back of the products in your bathroom cabinets. Here's a list of ingredients found in a well-known brand of men's face wash:

Water, sodium laureth sulfate, sodium chloride, cocamidopropyl hydroxysultaine, lauramidopropyl betaine, sodium cocoyl sarcosinate, tea-cocoyl glutamate, sodium hyaluronate, tocopheryl ethyl succinate ethyldimonium ethosulfate, sucrose, di-ppg-2 myreth-10 adipate, hexylene glycol, chamomilla recutita, butylene glycol, caprylyl glycol, cetyl triethylmonium dimethicone PEG-8 succinate, sodium sulfate, laureth-2, PEG-120 methyl glucose dioleate, EDTA, Disodium EDTA, Sodium Benzoate, Phenoxyethanol. And a toxic partridge in a pear tree.

Some of these compounds have been linked to reactions ranging from eczema to severe, life-threatening allergic reactions[11]. What's even more astonishing is that this product is not only perfectly legal, it has more than 70 online reviews averaging 4.8/5. Millions of men around the globe are subjecting themselves to these chemicals with an ignorant smile on their face.

Just because you don't experience an immediate reaction from a product does not mean that it causes you no harm. Some chemicals slowly change your body over many years, causing a lowering of testosterone, which can lead to cardiovascular disease and even suicidal tendencies[12].

It is my recommendation that unless you want to learn about all the ingredients in your bathroom, you throw out anything you don't understand and invest in an organic, plant-based range like *Sukin*, *Aesop* or *Dr Bronner's*. I use *Every Man Jack* deodorant, *Aubrey Organics* exfoliant and cologne, *Red Seal* toothpaste and *Sukin* for everything else.

If you want to take it a step further, live by the motto 'if you won't eat it, don't put it on your skin.' I have used activated charcoal as toothpaste, coconut oil as sun protection and hair wax; I've even used peppermint oil as a decongestant and mosquito bite relief. With a little education, you could completely transform the way you view your place in the natural world.

Healthy House, Healthy Body

How you clean yourself is important, but so is how you clean your house. Many of you might not be the one doing the cleaning, but I can assure you, the chemicals that remain on your kitchen top or in your freshly washed shirt are leaching into your body and causing damage. The safety of home-care products is even more loosely regulated than personal-care products. The chemicals in everyday residential laundry and cleaning staples are having a devastating effect on your health, and therefore your happiness.

Don't just take my word for it, take this every-day laundry powder ingredient list:

Sodium sulfate, sodium carbonate, sodium dodecylbenzene sulfonate, sodium silicate, sodium carbonate peroxide, zeolite, sodium acrylic acid/ma copolymer, c12-15 pareth-7, tetraacetyl ethylene diamine, perfume, disodium-anilino-morpholino-triazinyl-amino-stilbene-sulfonate, disodium distyrylbiphenyl disulfonate, cellulose gum, calcium sodium edtmp, phenylpropyl ethyl methicone, protease, amylase, mannanase, lipase, ci-74160.

Would you be comfortable sprinkling that over your kids?

What's the cheapest way to manufacture a cleaning product, and still make you think your home smells like a pine forest? Your home is one big science experiment, and you're the subject. Even if you feel like these products do a great job and it's worth the risk, would you risk the health of your child? With the knowledge you have now, would you subject your children to be a part of this experiment? Let's wait another 30 years and see the real effects of this ingredient list. With the current health trends, we can assume it won't be pretty.

Instead of handing over your dollars and your trust to these massive corporations, why not invest in more sustainable companies like *Earth Choice*, or refill your laundry products from a local health food store. As for cleaning your kitchen and bathroom, a simple combination of vinegar, baking soda, orange and eucalyptus oil will work perfectly 99 times out of 100 to kill bacteria, remove grease and bad odours.

Stop Microwaving Yourself

Further to cleaning products is the topic of electromagnetic frequency (EMF) radiation. The science is conclusive: chronic exposure to high amounts of EMF can cause significant harmful biological effects such as autoimmune conditions, chronic fatigue and even cancer[13,14,15]. The largest producers of EMF are WiFi routers, switch boards, mobile phones, power lines, solar power systems, and smart meters.

For us men, there have been many particularly alarming studies on the effects of cellphone radiation on our reproductive system. One of the most shocking sections of Tim Ferriss' book, *The 4-Hour Body*, included his experimentation with increasing sperm count and testosterone levels. Ferriss reported, "there were more than a handful of studies that showed significant decreases in serum testosterone in rats following even moderate exposure (30 minutes per day, five days a week, for four weeks) to 900 megahertz radio frequency electromagnetic fields (EMF), which is what most GSM cell phones produce"[16].

On a mission to increase his pitiful sperm count and testosterone levels, he removed his phone from his pocket for eleven weeks. Approximately nine weeks is required to generate new sperm cells, so he conservatively added a two-week buffer. The results from his self-experiment were startling[14]:

1. Ejaculate volume: 44% increase.
2. Motile sperm per milliliter: 100% increase.
3. Motile sperm per ejaculate: 185% increase.

Admittedly, this experiment was far from perfect, however these findings prompted me to immediately free my testicles from my mobile phone radiation once and for all. The risks far outweighed the benefits, and I vowed never to carry my phone in my pocket unless switched to airplane mode. Interestingly, the phantom vibrations on my left thigh vanished, and I have become much more aware of the heat and metallic sensations that arise from my digital devices. There's a chance that this is just an unfortunate consequence of subjective bias, but the reality is that high amounts of electromagnetic radiation can damage DNA[17], and so I now choose to avoid it as much possible. I'll take my virility over an email notification any day.

If you live in the city, you are likely bathing in a soup of radiation and may not fully realise the effect this is having on your body. If there are infants or children in your house, you need to be more cautious of EMF exposure due to their thinner skulls.

Although relocating from a high-rise apartment to an acreage in the country would be the easiest way to reduce your exposure to EMF, it's not always the most practical. Simple steps that you can take include:

1. Use an EMF blocking smartphone and tablet case such as *SafeSleeve*.
2. Never carry your phone in your pocket.
3. Use headphones for voice calls.
4. Use a *DefenderPad* laptop radiation shield when placing the computer directly on your body.
5. Turn off your WiFi router when not in use. Ideally you can connect directly via an ethernet cable when working on your laptop.
6. Switch your phone to airplane mode at night.

There are also EMF shielding underpants, and even whole body protection suits available online - but unless you want to run down the street shouting "THE SKY IS FALLING", then that might not be your style.

The Air We Breathe

Air quality has an enormous effect on our physiology. Imagine yourself trekking in the crisp forests of Tasmania or the untouched mountains of Patagonia, breathing the air deep into your lungs. The air is clean, vibrant, alive. You feel light, awake and energised. Now, recall how it feels to breathe in the most densely populated, concrete jungle you've experienced. Dusty, with fumes of petrol, deep fried food and human desperation. You feel just like your environment.

Fortunately, there are steps that you can take to reduce your exposure to toxic, poor quality air. Firstly, prioritise living near a trees (lots of them). Being across the road from a park, nursery, or a community garden is a good start. The further you can get out of the smog and pollution of the city and the closer to wilderness, the better the quality of air and the better your health. This seems obvious, but it is often overlooked when choosing your forever home.

Secondly, eliminate dampness and mould with good airflow, and if you live in an older home, use a dehumidifier. While living in Melbourne's winters, our dehumidifier would extract at least five litres of water from our bedroom every week. This excess dampness can lead to mould growth which can be highly toxic for some individuals. The science shows that mycotoxins (fungi) can cause allergies and food intolerances, genetic mutations, cognitive decline, and even autoimmune conditions.

The next step is to purify the air you live in. House plants are a very effective way to clean your air. There is a list online of NASA approved air-purifying plants that you can leave around your house. Depending on where you live, mother-in-law's tongues (no, it's a plant), or peace lilies are an excellent, easily maintained choice. In my opinion, you can never have e: greenery in your house; according to the University of I they can even improve your well-being by 47%[18].

It is possible to install a full home ducted air purifier systems with medical grade HEPA filters. This can get expensive, but it is worth it. Alternatively, if you're renting or planning to move in a couple of years, you can purchase a smaller, portable option like my *Blueair Sense* purifier. Within 30 seconds of turning this on, my bedroom feels cooler and clearer, and I leave it running whisper quiet all night.

One last method to pimp out the air in your home is with essential oils. Yep, the hippies were right. Using a simple, electric diffuser or flame burner, you can have your home smelling anyway you like, from vibrant blends of bergamot and lime to the sensual combination of ylang ylang and frankincense. Certain oils have differing effects on your neurochemistry[19,20]. Rosemary has been said to help with memory, orange and rose can alleviate depression, while the scent of lavender can help you calm down at night. I have been using oils for years to keep my home feeling light, fresh and clean. Incense can also work to this effect but some of the chemicals inside may be harmful, so I usually keep with essential oils. Go on, visit your nearest health food store or jump on www.iherb.com and give an organic essential oil a try.

Water, Water, Everywhere, Not a Drop to Drink

Finally, there is water. The water you drink, as well as bathe in, has a tremendous impact on your health. Water can be a vibrant, rich, life-giving fluid or it can be perished and polluted. Your body is mostly comprised of water, and so it makes sense that this would be true. When in harmony with nature, women's menstrual cycle is dictated by the moon due to the strong tidal pull that it holds[21]. Imagine yourself drinking from a freshwater stream in a cool, temperate rainforest high up on the mountainside. Now visualise tap water from your bathroom sink. Can you tell the difference?

In my apartment, I had a premium *Doulton Ultracarb* under-sink filter and a chrome *Sprite Kinetic Degradation Fluxion* (KDF) shower filter which cost less than $400 from www.psifilters.com.au. The options are endless for home filters. I would avoid reverse osmosis filtration systems unless the water is remineralised. As for alkaline water systems, there's no benefit to them, in fact, if anything they may be mildly detrimental due to the highly acidic environment of your stomach. If you are in your forever home, you should invest in an entire home water filtration system, which may cost $1,000 up to $10,000.

The purest place to source your water is from rain or natural springs. You can visit www.findaspring.com to show you any springs that are located nearby. You would need to take a few large glass jugs to the area and fill up. Although incredibly rewarding, venturing out into nature to gather water is not practical for most people unless you're big into 'rewilding'.

When my girlfriend and I moved into our apartment, she thought I was a little bit paranoid when buying a shower filter but after her first time under the tap, she immediately realised that she had been bathing in a chlorine gas chamber for nearly three decades. Her skin and hair felt softer than before, and she didn't experience a sluggish feeling from a hot shower. Every six months I change this filter, and it's shocking how much dirt and chemical filth is removed from the water we bathe in.

I have tried to keep this chapter as simple as possible to prevent an inundation of information. Any action to get you started on detoxing your home is better than inaction. There are so many choices available that it's sometimes hard to make any decision at all. Start by immediately removing all non-plant based personal and home-care products. Order yourself simple EMF protection devices online from earthingoz.com.au and turn off your WiFi and smartphones at night. Begin searching for providers of exceptional quality water filtration, whether it be an under sink or whole-house system.

The information I have given you is just the tip of the iceberg. There are entire books written on detoxing and maintaining a healthy home. *Is Your Home Making You Sick?* by Dr Peter Dingle and *The Healthy Home: Simple Truths to Protect Your Family from Hidden Household Dangers* by Dr Myron Wentz are two great places to learn how to reduce your exposure to environmental toxins.

You now have the knowledge you need to make your home a healthy place. The power is in your hands, and you can rest easy knowing that your home is safe for you, the environment and your family. With every step you take, you are getting closer to living in harmony with nature and ultimately yourself. Now get cleaning.

Chapter Six

Swim Like a Polar Bear, Bake Like a Snake

"It's not the strongest of the species that survives, nor the most intelligent. It is the one that is the most adaptable to change".

- *Charles Darwin*

Part of getting back to nature is exposing yourself to the elements. By changing up your environment, you provide your body with different stimuli that causes adaptation. These adaptations are usually positive, as in the case of the contents of this chapter. With challenge, there is growth, and what doesn't kill you makes you stronger. Of the elements of nature, none are more primal than heat and cold. Let's dive into the profoundly healing effects that heat and cold have had on my clients and myself.

The Sun produces many types of energy waves. One of them is far infrared energy; it's a wavelength of light that is longer than the visible spectrum. When it hits your skin, it directly vibrates and therefore heats the cells in your body.

Some amazing things happen when far infrared comes into contact with your body. Far infrared light stimulates enzymes in the mitochondria of your cells. These tiny organelles are the powerhouses of your body that create energy. By creating energy from light, one might argue that the human body is photosynthetic. In fact, it has been shown that this is exactly the case in the presence of chlorophyll from green plants[22]. This energy can be obtained from the sun or with the use of an infrared sauna.

When sitting in the sauna, a 'hyperthermic' effect occurs. This effect causes your heart to beat harder and faster, promoting blood flow and building cardiac strength. An article in the April 2009 issue of the Journal of Cardiology suggested that sauna therapy has shown profound benefits to patients with cardiovascular disease[23].

The infrared sauna can even promote the growth of new blood vessels to areas of low circulation, providing much needed oxygenated blood to undernourished tissues[24]. Those with previous injuries or aching joints usually experience pain relief from the increased circulation and anti-inflammatory effect.

Far infrared wavelengths directly penetrate the body tissues to a depth of nearly four cm. The cells that are exposed to this wavelength experience elevated growth and regeneration. Researcher Dr Rhonda Patrick is a huge advocate for the benefits of saunas. She suggests that heat acclimatisation is associated with massive increases in growth hormone and protein synthesis[25].

Collagen and elastin are two essential proteins of connective tissue that maintain their strength and elasticity. With an enhanced production of these proteins, the skin can begin to heal the degenerative change that happens over the course of ageing. Also, with frequent trips to the sauna, our tendons and ligaments become durable and flexible. An increase in protein synthesis also means more muscle growth for all of you striving to look and feel good naked.

The mild heat stress causes viruses and bacteria to be sensitized while your immune cells release powerful mechanisms that prime the body for better defence. After a few sessions, adaptation occurs due to the body's production of something called heat shock proteins, which increase antioxidant levels in the body[23].

Heat shock proteins arise due to the hormetic stress that the heat provides. Hormesis is a recovery process in which the body undergoes to adapt to a particular stimulus. The same thing occurs when we exercise, or drink the phytochemicals found in green tea. These hormetic responses have been shown to improve athletic performance, muscle growth, fat loss, the growth of new brain cells, improve learning and memory, and even increase longevity[23].

Exploring Cold Therapy

I first began taking regular cold showers after reading Tim Ferriss' *The 4-Hour Body*. Initially, it was difficult to submerge myself under the needle like iciness each morning, but soon I noticed some changes to my immune system and body composition. After a few months, I was the leanest I had ever been, and had significantly reduced hay fever symptoms. What was once a debilitating spring and summer affliction in the dry heat of Western Australia, my hay fever became barely noticeable. I was convinced.

Five years later, I was on The Great Ocean Road in southern Victoria in the middle of winter, sitting in a two degree ice bath, surrounded by 50 people at Wim Hof's first ever Australia retreat. I was quickly discovering that water conducts heat away from the body 25 times faster than air, and my physiology was changing rapidly. From the moment you step into your first ice bath, your whole body lights up, your breathing gets out of control, your testicles look for shelter in your mouth, and every cell in your body is screaming at you to get out. But you don't.

This is the moment that you exercise dominion over your mind. You begin to calm your breath and relax your body. You pick one crystal of ice and stare into it. You enter a state of calm and quiet. Everything else fades away including time itself. The power of the cold takes over.

On a physical level, cold therapy has been shown to[26,27]:

1. Boost positive dynorphin neurotransmitters such as noradrenaline and dopamine.
2. Treat depression.
3. Prevent neurodegenerative diseases and even damage from traumatic brain injury.
4. Elevate testosterone and growth hormone levels.
5. Increase metabolism, resulting in efficient fat loss.
6. Enhance fertility.
7. Increase strength and vitality.
8. Reduce inflammation and pain.

The mechanisms by which cold exposure affects the body are vast. For example, a rapid rise, sometimes five-fold, in the neurotransmitter norepinephrine, can dramatically reduce tumour necrosis factor alpha (TNF-alpha). TNF-alpha is a signalling protein which has been implicated in ageing, as well as almost every human disease ranging from type 2 diabetes, to inflammatory bowel disease, to cancer[26]. Not only does it suppress chronic inflammation, but regular cold water immersion has been shown to increase the number of white blood cells, particularly T lymphocytes, which fight off pathogens and cancer cells[26].

One of my clients, who runs a successful consulting organisation, is a frequent user of both infrared saunas and cold showers. After a few years of using the sauna twice per week, we began to deepen our conversation into cold showers. He had found the sauna to be quite cleansing and helped to 'get stuff out of him'. I encouraged him to give the cold showers a try as we were heading into winter. The next session he reported back with a feeling of invigoration, aliveness and he now starts every day under five degree water. After a few months of combining both cold showers and hot saunas, he now feels these tools help him become more aware and in tune with his body.

Convinced yet? Here's how to navigate the icy waters of cold immersion:

1. Place a stopwatch next to your shower where you can see it.
2. Begin by spending 10-30 seconds at the end of your hot shower with cold. Be sure to turn the hot water completely off as you need to go for that 'F*%k, that's icy!' feeling.
3. Increase the amount of time up to 120 seconds. At this point, most people don't even bother with the hot water beforehand.
4. Do this every morning for 28 days.
5. Buy a thermometer and 15-30 kg of ice.
6. Sit in a 5-degree ice bath for at least two minutes.
7. Shout expletives at your supportive bystanders/bemused pets.
8. Over several baths, you may slowly increase the length of time to 10 minutes.
9. Gradually add more ice and reduce the temperature to below two degrees.
10. Dance in celebration like a viking, for you have conquered the cold.

Before an ice bath, it's helpful to perform three to five rounds of the Wim Hof Method. However, you should never perform any breath techniques under or inside a body of water without supervision. When lying in the ice, keep your hands on your thighs and control your breath. I repeat, control your breath.

Heart attacks and permanent nerve damage are real potential dangers, so please confirm with medical supervision to confirm whether you are healthy enough to practice this section of the program. Don't be alarmed if your doctor looks at you in bewilderment.

We humans typically seek comfort, particularly physical comfort, as much as possible. When we succumb to this need for comfort, we prevent ourselves from growth. There is a concept called voluntary discomfort, that is a choice in which you take the uncomfortable route simply because it fosters growth, makes you a stronger, tougher person. Exercise is a form of voluntary discomfort for most people. In 2016, I chose to sell my car, and instead carry 15-20 kg of groceries on my back each week. It was a lot easier to drive to the whole foods store, but I feel a lot more rewarded when I open the front door with a mountain of food on my back. In a primal sense, it feels like I am bringing home the hunt.

I want to encourage you to entertain the idea of voluntary discomfort. Our life is filled with more pleasures than it ever has been, and we are becoming immune to it. The more pleasures we seek, often the less happy we become. Some cultures with just enough for food, water and shelter are some of the most content people on the planet because their rewards from their efforts are so tangible and the rest of the time they focus on relationships with family and friends.

So next time you have the option to walk, bike or take public transport instead of drive, do so. If you can, make use of a sweat lodge or sauna, breathe through the discomfort of the heat. And next time you hop in the shower, take the blue pill. There will be no turning back.

Chapter Seven

Japanese Wisdom

"Look deep into nature, and then you will understand everything better".

- *Albert Einstein*

In the early 1980s, a radical idea was put forth to the country of Japan that would revolutionise their health care philosophy. This proposal was so far-out that it took over 15 years for medical journals to catch up. It would be one of the greatest discoveries in preventative medicine of all time. This radical concept is known as forest bathing. It seems like common sense, but forest bathing, otherwise known as shinrin-yoku, which translates to "taking in the forest atmosphere", is now medically recognised as having profoundly healing effects on human physiology[28,29]. That's right, spending time in nature is good for you. Some of the significant healing effects of shinrin-yoku include:

1. Reduced cortisol levels[30].
2. Improved sight and hearing[31].
3. Boosting the immune system[31].
4. Reducing pulse rate and blood pressure[29].
5. Reducing cerebral hyperactivity[29].
6. Improved focus and concentration[29].
7. Decreased inflammation[31].
8. Improved sleep[30].
9. Increased pain tolerance[31].

The above list of benefits nearly includes - either directly or indirectly - most physiological processes in the body. There is likely not one part of you that does not benefit from spending time in nature. Let's dive a little deeper into why this might be the case by exploring what happens to your body when you take in the forest air.

When we gaze amongst clouds, the ocean, rustling leaves or toward a campfire, our eyes tend to dance from one unfocused frame of motion to another. Staring upon these natural phenomena is mesmerising. How many times have you been able to stare into the world of fire for minutes on end without blinking? The reason for this is because your eyes cannot focus, and the muscles that control your eye's lens can relax, which also allows your brain activity to slow down. A reduction in brain waves has been shown to improve cognitive function and concentration and lead to greater feelings of happiness[32].

The natural world is loudest during the morning inside a rain forest at about 32 decibels. If you've ever woken up deep in the jungles of Asia or Latin America, you would know how terrifyingly loud this can be. Even more terrifying is that most anthropogenic (human-made) noises, especially in cities, are between 80-120 decibels. This noise is many times louder than our ears have evolved with and can lead to chronic cortisol overload and hypertonic muscles. This can create an excessively tight jaw and abdomen, and somewhat more obviously, permanent hearing damage[31].

When walking in the forest, there is that distinct smell of living, breathing plant biosphere. One of these smells is a group of chemicals known as phytoncides. Plants produce phytoncides to ward off insects, but science has discovered that these natural 'pesticides' actually enhance the functions of our immune system, specifically our natural killer cells[28]. Just 12-hours spent in the forest can increase the number of natural killer cells in circulation for up to 7 days afterwards[29]. These immune cells are known for fighting off cancerous and precancerous cells. There are also immune boosting parasites and bacteria that thrive on the living matter of trees and in the dirt.

The immune regulating effects continue. While walking in the forest, our body reduces the number of pro-inflammatory cytokines such as interleukin-6 (IL-6) and TNF-alpha[29]. Chronically elevated levels of these cytokines, or chemical messengers, are associated with chronic inflammatory conditions such as rheumatoid arthritis and multiple sclerosis.

Taking it a step further, there is the option to get slightly more intimate with nature via barefoot walking. You would likely do this on the beach, but in the forest, it's much rarer to see someone take off their hiking boots and trudge through the woods. After all, there are snakes, and it is *terribly* dirty.

Unfortunately though, you're not allowing your feet to connect directly with the earth. This connection between foot and floor is where an exchange of electrons occurs. Through the normal physiological process, our body builds up an increased level of electromagnetic charge[31]. In tribal times, we were connected with the planet every day, however, in today's culture, we sometimes don't get to dump our electromagnetic waste into the earth for a whole day.

In fact, many apartment dwellers in busy cities may not touch their skin with an earthed structure for days on end. Placing your palms and feet on the bare earth can have a tremendously calming effect on your nervous system. This process is known as earthing and has been shown to reduce inflammation, and chronic stress as well as improves sleep and pain tolerance[31].

While growing up in the sunny, active, beachside city of Perth, Western Australia, I would spend the majority of my time outside, totally barefoot. I developed strong skin and muscles on my feet and ankles and grew connected with the earth. I moved to the inner-city Melbourne suburb of Fitzroy, Victoria, where there isn't a beach for many kilometres, and let's just say it's a little more 'grunge'. Over time my feet became soft and weak, and I had lost much of my connection with nature. Now on trips outside the city, I relish in every opportunity I can to take my shoes off and walk on the bare earth. I encourage you to do the same.

If getting your feet dirty is not your thing, there are sandals called *Earth Runners* that allow a direct connection between the earth and your feet. To understand this for yourself, next time you are at a picnic in the park or walking on the beach barefoot, pay close attention to how you feel. You may realise a deeper connection to your humanness.

New information will continue to emerge, which tells us that interacting with the biosphere is beneficial to our health. For example, the sun gives us vitamin D, but you can't just take a vitamin D pill and get all of the benefits of the sun. This is because particular types of UV radiation also decrease inflammation, and your risk for demyelinating diseases like multiple sclerosis[31]. Conversely, when we expose ourselves to chilly weather, our body reacts by contracting the muscles in our skin and the blood vessels beneath. This is the feeling of being alive.

We don't yet know all the benefits of interacting with nature. From the warmth of the sun, the cold of the wind, the water, or the complete orchestra of nature's sounds, there are so many possible encounters that your body can have with biology. As eco-biomechanist, Katy Bowman says, "We are missing out on an unquantifiable number of interactions with nature, and our physiology is the worse for it"[31].

I once stood knee deep in the surf of Bondi Beach, New South Wales, Australia, for 20 minutes. I was amongst a group of movement students with the renowned teacher, Ido Portal. We were instructed to stare out into the ocean and try not to move a muscle. "Don't blink, don't even swallow," I remember him saying. As we stood there gazing out onto the crashing waves, time began to disintegrate. I became acutely aware of every sensation of my body from the sounds of kids playing off in the distance, to the sand collapsing beneath my feet. Tears began to fall down my face, and I felt a deep sense of peace wash over me. Nature had taken me in.

I want you to follow the way. I want you to spend more time in nature. Our evolution as humans has seen us develop biological benefits from the flora around us, and we are denying its benefits by distancing ourselves from it. If you live in the city, put it on your calendar to take a few hours on the weekend to venture out to the forest, to the beach or a mountaintop. This reconnection should happen at least once per month. Leave your phone at home or in the car. Go alone, or with friends or family. Take off your shoes and look up at the sky and smile. This is the mysterious phenomenon called life. It is all around you, and it is incredibly healing. All you need to do is engage with it.

Chapter Eight

Rhythm is a Dancer

"Even a soul submerged in sleep is hard at work and helps make something of the world".

- Heraclitus, Fragments

Everything in nature follows rhythms and cycles. From the sun rising and setting, to the seasons of the year, and even the earth's electromagnetic frequency. Well, the human body is no different. A major key to health is our circadian rhythm or the sleep-wake cycle.

The circadian rhythm is a 24 hour cycle in the physiological process of all living beings. This cycle is regulated by the master circadian pacemaker in the suprachiasmatic nucleus of the brain[33], which then commands the hormones of the rest of the body, primarily produced from the brain and adrenal glands. These crucial hormones include DHEA, cortisol, and melatonin. Our body has an inbuilt clock, but this can be manipulated by light, temperature and other biological phenomena such as electromagnetic fields.

We have evolved to fall asleep just after sunset and wake up just before sunrise, however in today's modern world, this normal rhythm has been altered, and we either don't achieve the right *type* of sleep or don't obtain the right *amount* of sleep. My belief is that 80% of optimal performance is rest and recovery.

Sleep regulates about 15-20% of your entire genome, meaning your genes can turn on or off with sufficient levels of sleep. When you deplete your body of sleep over the long term, you can experience severe ill effects ranging from lethargy and depression, to psychosis and death[34]. Sleep is no joke!

Research has shown that a minimum of seven to eight hours is required for optimal brain function, sex hormone production, fat loss and prevention of certain diseases such as cardiovascular disease and diabetes[34]. In fact, a study of 531 men showed that males who sleep for four hours produce 60% less testosterone than men who sleep eight hours[35]. That means the entrepreneur with that die-hard, spartan-like mentality who proclaim "sleep is for the weak", is twice as weak, masculinity-speaking, as their sleepy, sloth-like brothers.

To give you an idea of the importance of a proper functioning circadian rhythm, the timetable below represents this cycle in your daily existence.

06:45   Sharpest rise in cortisol and blood pressure.
07:30   Light causes melatonin secretion to stop.
08:30   Gut motility increases.
09:00   Highest testosterone secretion.
10:00   High alertness.
14:30   Best coordination.
15:30   Fastest reaction time.
17:00   Greatest cardiovascular efficiency and muscle strength. Peak in protein synthesis.
18:30   Highest blood pressure.
19:00   Leptin released (fatty acid metabolism) and insulin falls. Highest body temperature.
21:00   Melatonin secretion starts (if in three to four hours of darkness).
22:30   Bowel movements suppressed.
23:00   Brain-gut connection quiets down.

00:00	Melatonin peaks - Leptin and Thyroid hormones up to regulate and induces fat loss. Prolactin release increases cell autophagy and growth hormone release.
02:00	Deepest sleep. Nervous system repair and growth.
04:30	Lowest body temperature. Peak fat burning efficiency and peak immune function.

Let's break this down in more practical detail.

Firstly, if you're not well and truly in a deep sleep by 2 a.m., you are not able to repair and grow new brain cells. This means learning will grind to a halt and brain ageing occurs at a much faster rate.

If you haven't been asleep for at least 6 hours by 4:30 a.m., your fat burning will be significantly reduced, and you will have a compromised immune system.

By 6:45 a.m. you should be waking up naturally, depending on the seasons and which latitude you call home, of course. In winter you will require more sleep, in summer less.

By 8:30 a.m., you should have eaten breakfast and eliminated yesterday's.

At 9:30 a.m. our testosterone is now elevated along with your level of alertness, so if you're able to, now is a good time to exercise.

However between 2:30 p.m. and 5 p.m., you will heighten levels of performance characteristics such as strength, coordination and reaction time, so this is also an effective time to move your body.

The hormonal situation at 7 p.m. indicates that it's best to not eat after this time if fat loss is your priority.

By 9 p.m., you should be well and truly beginning to wind down, but this will only happen if you're avoiding artificial light.

Although you may be asleep by 10 p.m., if you were watching TV right beforehand, your sleep will not be as deep, or restorative had you been reading a book under candlelight for two hours prior.

For optimal gut function, appetite regulation, and peak fat loss efficiency, being asleep by 11 p.m. is critical. If you're interested in anti-aging, recovery and reducing inflammation, then midnight is when these functions occur, providing that you've been asleep for a few hours already.

I'm sure that from the above description of your circadian rhythm, sleep is incredibly important for you to thrive as a human being. How then do we ensure optimal sleep patterns while living the life of a modern man? Big screens, little screens, and email beeps all get in the way.

Let's take a deep dive into the Top 15 Sleep Strategies to help you get your best night's sleep since you were a baby.

1. Sleep in a completely dark, cold(ish) room. This helps the release of melatonin, the hormone that is responsible for the secretion all other hormones that promote deep sleep and repair.

2. Meditate before bed. Just 5-10 minutes of deep, focused breathing can be sufficient to decrease cortisol and wind down. There are plenty of smartphone apps such as Headspace, Omvana and Calm that bring you guided meditations to have a restful sleep.

3. Turn off all mobile and WiFi signals. This includes turning your phone off or on airplane mode. The EMF can disrupt the body's normal sleep cycle. Particularly if you have young

children, make sure you turn off the signals emitting from your Wi-Fi router. Some people are more sensitive to EMF radiation than others.

4. If you need an alarm, use an app like *Sleep Cycle*. This app measures your sleep patterns and only sounds during your most awake state within a given 30 minute period. It's very effective at eliminating the lightning-bolt-to-the-heart sensation that a regular phone alarm brings, allowing for a happier and more peaceful morning.

5. Avoid blue light two hours before bed. If you must work until late, use the computer software *F.lux*, night shift mode on your smartphone, or even take the next step and purchase some blue-light blocking glasses. It's also important to consider the lighting in your house. Choose warm LEDs with the lowest lux possible, particularly in your bathroom and toilet, as these areas will be used right before bed.

6. Avoid social media and television before bed. These mediums stimulate dopamine. Chronic use can lead to dopamine resistance and depression. They are also incredibly unfulfilling. Instead, talk to your partner or read your children a bedtime story. If you live alone, read yourself a bedtime story.

7. Move. Exercise is one of the best tools to help regulate circadian rhythm and improve your quality of sleep. Ancient man wasn't known for being a couch potato.

8. Eat. Make sure you eat plenty of food. I find that poor sleep is one of the first indicators that my clients aren't eating enough food. Carbohydrates like rice or potatoes are very efficient at reducing evening cortisol levels and ensuring a good night's sleep. Eating first thing resets your circadian clock and tells your body "Hey, it's morning, wake up!". Hence breakfast, breaking the fast, it's time to be alive again.

9. Take a cold shower before bed. This one is counter-intuitive but has been shown to promote melatonin production[36].

10. Sleep on a firm, organic futon mattress like the ones from *Samina* or *Organature*. These beds are free from carcinogenic flame retardants and other industrial chemicals. You don't want to breathe these chemicals in for eight hours every night for 10 years. A futon mattress promotes well-being of your spine and joints, as there is no *Posturepedic* nonsense to cast your body into an unnatural position. Plus, the ability to sleep on the floor without a pillow makes camping that much more luxurious.

11. Use a pulsed electromagnetic field (PEMF) therapy device like the *EarthPulse*. During my irregular working hours as a personal trainer, I suffered from anxious sleeping patterns. I would wake up in a panic in the middle of the night, feeling like I have missed my alarm. This device simulates the earth's magnetic rhythms and was one of the most useful tools to help me get to sleep immediately. I believe it's essential if you're in a high-rise apartment or surrounded by EMF radiation. I also found that I always began to wake up right before my alarm sounded, which really helps you feel on top of your day before it starts.

12. Use an air purifier, like the *Blueair Sense* from Denmark. This brings a noticeable difference to the quality of air in your bedroom.

13. Listen to binaural beats or nature sounds. These help to reduce cortisol as well as the frequency of your brain waves. A gradual slide from beta to delta is much more healing than an immediate crash into an unconscious coma after working all day. During one particularly stressful week, I took my client, Vince, to a consult room, turned off the lights and placed my headphones in his ears with my *Brainwaves* app. As he lay there, listening to the sounds, I guided him through 15 minutes of

rebalancing breath work. His worries of life began to dissoi.
and he started smiling in a barely conscious state by the end.
In his case, this was much better for his general health than
smashing him with deadlifts and pushups for an hour.

14. Use supplements:

1. Magnesium - Take 10-20 mg/kg body weight (800-
    1600 mg for an 80 kg man), depending on your difficulty
    of sleeping.
2. Passion flower extract - 1 ml dropper on the tongue can
    prevent you from waking up throughout the night.
3. Phenibut - a herb that promotes gamma-aminobutyric
    acid (GABA) production in the brain. Only use this
    for a period of four to eight weeks during particularly
    stressful times as the body can develop a dependence.

15. Get plenty of exposure to the natural rhythms of the earth.
From watching the sunset and sunrise, to walking barefoot on
grass, getting in tune with the Earth's circadian rhythm is very
effective at improving sleep, particularly if you are experiencing
jet lag.

Suffering from poor quality sleep is one of the most common
complaints that I hear from my clients. To me, it's no surprise
given we've become so far removed from the natural rhythm
of our tribal ancestors. There are no more sessions of storytelling by the campfire after a big feast. Instead, we have dinner
well after sunset and essentially use our phones to shine a little
flashlight into our retinas until right before we fall asleep.
We don't eat properly, and so our blood glucose levels swing
wildly throughout the night. And we're in a state of such high
stress that we continue to think about work for our last waking
moments. That email about project X that you have to send to
client Y should not be costing you your health.

It is essential to maximise your quality of sleep to improve the quality of your life. I want you to implement just five strategies that I have outlined in this chapter. Choose ones that you've done in the past and worked for you, or try something new entirely. With these tips and tricks, you should be able to achieve at least 7 hours of unbroken sleep each night, and that means no trips to the toilet either! You have spent enough time prioritising your productivity. It's time to start prioritising your recovery to ensure you can keep your output high for another few decades. Work hard. Take rest. You deserve it.

Part Two: Nature - Summary

Create a home that's healthy for you and the planet.

1. Use only organic cleaning products and toiletries.
2. Consider the quality of your air and water.
3. Keep your phone away from your vital organs.

Expose yourself to the elements.

4. Experiment with consistent use of saunas.
5. Commit to daily cold showers for two minutes.

Get back to your roots.

6. Take at least one day per month to spend immersed in nature.
7. Use this time with family and friends or alone in self-reflection.

Optimise your sleep.

8. Make it your goal to reclaim your circadian rhythm using the Top 15 Sleep Strategies.

nutrition

Chapter Nine

The One Diet to Rule Them All

"You have brains in your head. You have feet in your shoes. You can steer yourself in any direction you choose".

- Dr Seuss

The quest has been going on for decades. The search for the optimal way of eating for human beings to thrive has given birth to a lot of new scientific discoveries, and we now know more nuances about human biology than ever. So it makes sense then, that we'd be at least *close* to uncovering the ultimate human diet.

Well, the truth is that this one and only, complete way to eat does not exist. No, not even pizza. The optimal way for you to eat depends entirely on who you are, where you come from and what has happened to you up until this very moment. The search all over the globe from the Australian Aborigines to Greenlandic Inuits has revealed a diverse range of foods that allow this human animal to flourish, depending on the climate of the environment and genetic makeup of our DNA.

For example, indigenous food sources for Greenlandic Inuits includes sea and land mammals, birds and fish, and in the warmer months, seaweeds, tubers and some berries. A traditional diet in Papua New Guinea also includes seafood but much more fruits, coconuts and tropical vegetables such as cassava. The caloric intake for Inuits was predominantly animal fats and proteins, however, for the Papua New Guinean culture, a much larger percentage is made of carbohydrates, particularly fructose.

This investigation into nutritional genomics allows us to determine which foods may work better for you. I've seen this in practice: An Asian man may tolerate up to 500g white rice per day, but give him the same amount of potato, and he may blow up like a puffer fish. His body does not like it because for thousands of years, he wasn't eating it.

Before coaching at 5EW, I was following a high fat, low carb diet because of all the experts and cherry-picked research supporting this way of eating. It wasn't until I learnt that my body type was in fact very carbohydrate tolerant, that I began eating an obscene amount of carbs and felt the benefits immediately. Upon eating 400g white rice or 600g sweet potato each day, I started sleeping properly, recovering from training faster and my body composition improved.

The opposite is also true. I have worked with others who only sniff a carbohydrate molecule and begin putting on body fat. They may have some form of insulin resistance or unhealthy gut microbiome and the sugars and fibres in even the healthiest of carbohydrate rich foods interact badly with their internal biochemistry.

My point is that there is no one-size-fits-all approach to nutrition. We have to take a personalised look at what you eat and sometimes even how you eat it. The media can release an article outlining that meat consumption causes cancer, but there are just as many arguments as to why meat consumption may prevent cancer, such as an increase in amino acids to assist in white blood cell function and liver detoxification.

Let's look at a few typical eating habits and see who they might suit best.

Ketogenic diets are relatively new in mainstream media. The consumption of high fat, moderate protein and low carbohydrate foods assists in the production of ketones, which can be used as a fuel source, much like glucose. The argument is that ketones are a much more sustainable source of energy and have been shown to alleviate symptoms in chronic inflammatory and neurological conditions such as diabetes, learning disabilities and epilepsy. The Inuit diet would be classified as ketogenic and was believed to keep them warm, strong and even healthy, especially during the colder months.

I first began experimenting with a ketogenic diet in late 2013 and initially found very positive effects. I could concentrate for hours on end with laser-like focus and found it very easy to reduce body fat. One of the benefits of a ketogenic diet is that you don't have uncontrolled fluctuations in blood sugar levels, which means you're less likely to have brain fog, irritability and body fat storage.

For most readers, this type of eating would work very efficiently for at least three months, providing that you consume enough calories. Be forewarned, if you eliminate carbohydrates and restrict protein without increasing your level of fat intake, you will only feel lethargic and tired, which believe it or not, are very appropriate symptoms of being underfed.

It's very unnatural to have spoonfuls of coconut oil or ghee from grass-fed cattle on top of your meals. It can even make some people go to the toilet rather abruptly if your digestive system is not used to the high consumption of fats. I remember in my early health evangelism days; I poisoned my Dad for an entire day with a high-fat smoothie. The porcelain was never the same again.

As I mentioned before, high fat, low carbohydrate diets can work wonders for people with an overgrowth of gut bacteria or poor blood glucose management. If you are over 20% body fat, this will likely be you to some degree. One of the major drawbacks for this diet is that it can leave the nervous system excessively stimulated. So if you are chronically stressed, overstimulated or have trouble sleeping, this is probably not an appropriate long-term solution.

High carb diets have been around for a very long time. Traditional cultures in Africa and Northern America even used pure honey as their primary fuel source for some parts of the year. A modern high carbohydrate diet however, is vastly different to a traditional version. Today's high carb foods are pizza, pasta, bread, spreads, pastries, etc. These foods contain not only a high amount of carbohydrates, but more importantly, contain a very large amount of inflammatory products such as gluten, processed dairy, sugar and farming chemicals.

Unfortunately, these toxic food chemicals have positioned all carbohydrates as demonic and deadly. The reality is that many men, particularly those who are leaner in body shape and under a high degree of stress perform much better with carbohydrates in their diet.

Take Ben for example. Ben was a huge ketone advocate. Like myself, he learned about ketogenic diets online and believed it was for everyone. He was regularly measuring his blood glucose and ketone levels. Surprisingly, as a very fit father of a three-year-old son and running a personal training business, he couldn't get his blood glucose levels below 6 mmol/L. By conservative estimates, this is pre-diabetic. When recommended to drop the high-fat lifestyle and instead consume significant amounts of carbohydrates at night, Ben's morning glucose levels dropped to between 4.0-4.5. He has since put on a stack of muscle and feels unstoppable.

Unlike the ketogenic diet, a high-carb diet is recommended for men who are very active and below 20% body-fat. Carbohydrate consumption raises blood glucose, causing a rise in the hormone insulin. This hormone suppresses our primary stress hormone, cortisol, in turn making us calm and sleepy. It's no wonder Spanish and Italian cultures have a 2 p.m. snooze every afternoon post-carbohydrate feast.

Best friend to the ketogenic craze is intermittent fasting. Fat as fuel is much more sustainable and can work well with intermittent fasting, otherwise, know as time-restricted feeding. You restrict your eating window to between 6 to 12 hours, or you could fast for one to two entire days each week. Fasting is a form of hormetic stress and is practised all over the world, primarily for spiritual reasons. The longevity and cognitive enhancing effects are well researched, and fasting is becoming increasingly popular. I have tried it and have used it with some of my clients. As busy, over-stimulated individuals, they do enjoy a break from eating but often find their sleep patterns suffer and their body composition stalls after a few weeks.

If pushed too far, fasting can be detrimental to your health due to excessive cortisol stimulation. I feel comfortable with a 12-hour eating window, to ensure I receive the benefits of autophagy (cellular rubbish removal) without over-stressing my body.

At opposing ends of the dietary spectrum are Paleo and Veganism. One believes animal-based foods are the only way to eat and the other believes that meat is murder and honey is slavery. The most difficult time of a discussion on nutrition is when emotion and belief systems get in the way of biological facts.

It's true some people can be insanely strong, virile and vegan. As my colleague pointed out that most successful long-term vegans are male, have excellent carbohydrate tolerance and likely have longer digestive tracts. This is an evolutionary biological trait that allows their bodies to cope with the increased level of sugars and fibres found in plant-based foods. As for the male component of a successful vegan, I can only suspect that females are more susceptible to the adverse effects of a reduced fat intake, which disrupts their delicate balance of sex hormones.

In my own experience, I have never coached a successful vegan and have only seen a handful online that make this dietary choice work. If you are interested in exploring the ecological, environmental, spiritual and biological consequences of Veganism or Vegetarianism, the most well-researched book I have read is *The Vegetarian Myth*, written by Lierre Keith, who was a vegan for, in her words, "21 hauntingly painful years".

Weston A. Price wrote the book *Nutrition and Physical Degeneration*. As a dentist, he travelled the globe in the early 1900s to identify traditional diets. He saw a lot of dental decay in England at the time and noticed people who ate closer to their natural habitat had less damage to their teeth and bone structures. These people were consuming high amounts of local plants and animal products, particularly foods made up of protein and fat.

Since then, it's been widely reported that no traditional cultures have ever adopted an entirely vegan diet. The oldest known vegetarian culture is the Indian Yogis. This group was primarily based on agriculture and consumed pulses (legume seeds), grains, dairy, and eggs. Keep in mind that this group of people were spending most of their days exploring the non-physical, not supporting a family or managing a sales team.

Around my 21st birthday, I came across a book entitled *Deep Nutrition* by Dr Catherine Shanahan. This book was my first exposure to ancestral eating. Bone broths, offal and fermented foods were never a part of my diet growing up, and this book was showing me that these foods were not only making people healthier but also more beautiful. Based on geometric calculations of facial bone formations, cultures who ate these foods over generations experienced fewer deformations and diseases that are suffered so commonly by developed nations[37]. They also showed more facial symmetry and were more attractive[38].

It seems to me that the closer to the food source we manage to place ourselves, the more likely we are to make decisions that are conducive to optimal health for us and the planet. I have recently been getting interested in hunting and gathering and after much research, I believe that this is the way we're supposed to eat. The history of our relationship with nature is hundreds of thousands of years old. The oldest known agricultural tradition is in Turkey, only about 10,000 years ago. Keep in mind Homo sapiens have been around 300,000 years; to go against our ancestral way of being is to go against hundreds of thousands of years of evolution with the planet.

If all this discussion leaves you overwhelmed, I have a few questions for you to ask yourself that will help you determine if your diet is on the right track.

1. How is my physical energy? From the ability to which you can exercise hard without injury, to the quality of your libido, your diet significantly impacts the energy that you carry yourself with throughout the day.

2. Do I experience food cravings? Sugar cravings are heavily linked to a deficiency in certain trace minerals such as chromium and zinc. So before you feel like your body is telling you it needs sugar, question if you are eating enough nutrient dense foods. In my own experience, sweet cravings can be a direct result of hypoglycaemia (low glucose levels), which may be caused by simply not eating enough food.

3. How sustained am I an hour after meals? If I ever have a

breakfast of muesli and fruit, I will be ravenous in less than two hours. This is because meals high in protein and fat promote sensitivity to the hormone leptin which signals to our brain that we are full and consequently, we lose body fat.

4. How is my mental clarity? This is a big one for you. Is your afternoon performance at work being impeded by that muffin and chai cinnamon sprinkle latte you had for breakfast?

5. What is the quality of my emotional well-being? Too often we can link stress to our job or relationships, but we cannot forget there is a huge nutritional connection. Deficiencies in certain amino acids such as tryptophan can drastically alter our sleep and emotional state. Don't let your nutritional ignorance determine the quality of your relationships and working potential.

6. Am I at my ideal body composition? In other words, using no-one else's measures but your own, ask yourself, "Do I feel good naked?".

If the answer is no or unsatisfactory to any of the preceding questions, then take that as feedback for you to make a change. There is an old saying: One man's food is another man's poison. What's right for you at this point in your life may be different to your colleague or your partner.

What's more, your diet will even need to change throughout your life. As an infant you were suckling 10-15 times per day, however as you head into your senior years, you may only eat two to three large meals in a 24-hour period. Depending on your age, physical activity and state of your health, your dietary needs will change. Fasting may be beneficial for you for a few months or years, but don't be so attached to your dietary lifestyle that you cannot see when your food is no longer working for you. Ultimately, there is no one diet to rule them all. Nutrition must be personal, and it's important that you pay attention to your body's sophisticated feedback mechanisms. Too often in our culture, we have outsourced our intuition to the latest research. But always remember, your body's wisdom is your best form of medicine. If you're feeling sub-par at anytime, just go through the above checklist. It's up to you to get back in touch with that innate intelligence.

Chapter Ten

It's What You Don't Do That Counts

"I really regret eating healthy today".

- *No one, ever.*

It seems to me that the older someone becomes, the more likely they are to tout the youth-enhancing effects of an exotic, barely pronounceable food. I've been in the health and fitness industry long enough to see superfoods come and go; almost all have had less effect on people's internal biochemistry than a sneeze from a tickle.

We're all searching for that fountain of youth food that will keep us bouncing on trampolines past a century, but most of the time this addiction just feeds the pockets of food manufacturing companies. I'm less concerned about how many goji berries and kale leaves that you eat and believe it's much more important to consciously select what you *don't* eat.

For the first four weeks of every new member's journey at 5EW, they undertake a *Fresh Start*. Kind of like a reboot for their entire body, this four to six week program eliminates all inflammatory foods, and floods the body with nutrient dense foods. It's designed (for the time being) to get the person to switch from using carbohydrates as a fuel source to fat and amino acids.

A crude analogy of food fuel sources goes like this: Carbohydrates are the twigs and kindling you place on top of a fire, and fats are the big heavy logs that slowly burn for hours, providing heat for the whole family. The exception to this analogy is that this fire actually works best when you use the logs before the kindling.

So we switch fuel sources, eliminate inflammatory foods, and provide copious amounts of nutrients to heal the body quickly. Some of the transformations we see are astounding. Bearing in mind that we ask these people to eat as much as possible - sometimes twice as much as they have been eating for years - it's not uncommon to see a loss of 3-5% body fat and gain of 2-3 kg lean muscle. Not only do they look better with their shirt off, but their cheeks and chin have shrunk, their skin is clearer and tighter, they're sleeping much better, and their energy is through the roof. It's one of my favourite things to see someone after this four week period for their first reassessment. "The system works", I always say.

So what foods do we eliminate? Let's go through them one by one.

Pasteurised, homogenised, conventional milk, cream and cheese. I call this white water with some rancid sugars, proteins and fats. The reasons to eliminate conventional dairy are vast, but for brevity, we want to reduce inflammation. I've never met someone who has eliminated these foods and not reported better cognition, clearer airways or smoother digestion. Organic butter and ghee are excellent; organic goats cheese in moderation.

Soy is one of the best cons of the superfood industry. What better way to earn insane profits than by selling one of the cheapest foods marketed to upper-middle class, yoga tight-wearing, vegan mums. Soy used to be an industrial chemical, and it's now in your latte. The phytoestrogens disrupt sex-hormones in the body, leading to vegan and vegetarian mothers being five times more likely to give birth to boys with severe sexual dysfunction, such as a shorter anogenital space[39]. Some young girls have had to go through puberty at eight years old after being fed soy based formula as an infant[39]. Other potential terrors of soy include high amounts of phytic acid, trypsin inhibitors, goitrogens and saponins, which can lead to thyroid dysfunction, cognitive decline, digestive issues, malnutrition and even cancer[39]. For further reading, get *The Whole Soy Story* by Dr Kaayla T. Daniel.

Sugar is commonly known as toxic, but still, people eat it. That's because it's in nearly every single type of processed food, from curry paste to mayonnaise, to bread and deli meats. It's also one of the most addictive substances on the planet. Your evolutionary biology says that when you come across some berries, you must gorge. It's an incredibly efficient source of energy and is usually accompanied by many nutrients. However today's sugar laden foods are anything but nutrient dense, and your evolutionary brain will still tell you to eat as much as possible. The dopamine surge in your brain is much like that of a cocaine addict and in fact, many tout that sugar may be more addictive than cocaine[37].

Artificial colours, flavours and sweeteners are a no-brainer. Studies have been emerging since the early 2000s indicating these toxic synthetic chemicals cause a myriad of problems, from behavioural disorders to cancer[40]. Don't touch them.

Grains include wheat, barley, rye, oats, white rice, brown rice, black rice, red rice, farro, corn, millet, and to some degree buckwheat, amaranth and quinoa. All grains are carbohydrate rich, fat-free, low-protein foods that require a significant amount of processing and cooking to be edible for human consumption. This makes most grains difficult to digest properly and can cause problems with blood sugar management[39]. Grains are also one of the most heavily sprayed agricultural nightmares, so be sure to get your grains from an organic or biodynamic source.

The last three that I mentioned are pseudo-cereals and in fact come from seeds, but constitute a similar nutrient profile and require a similar method of processing. After the 5EW *Fresh Start*, many people can tolerate these pseudo-cereals and rice. I almost always recommend men consume carbohydrates, including potatoes and sweet potatoes after strength training or at dinner. The number of carbohydrates depends on body fat density.

Gluten is another nightmare food that most people wish did not exist. Particularly in Australia, we have one of the highest populations of gluten intolerance in the world[39]. For easier (and cheaper) harvesting, the crops are sprayed with immense amounts of glyphosate or Round-Up one week before machinery grinds them up. As for the organic certification, in this economy, I don't believe it has much merit. Gluten containing foods are also terrible for the environment. Mono-crop cultures from soy, to corn, to wheat, have decimated topsoil due to herbicides and insecticides, which fuels global warming while destroying plant and animal biodiversity[39].

The protein in gluten, called gliadin, increases intestinal permeability in every person that eats it. This intestinal permeability, or leaky gut, has been linked to our current epidemic of allergies, autoimmune conditions and neurodegenerative diseases[41]. If you're not convinced, eliminate it for four weeks and see if you look and feel healthier. Not everyone is allergic to it, but every person I have coached is intolerant of it.

Legumes are another polarising food group. The purpose of eliminating this food group is to ease digestion and ultimately reduce inflammation. Legumes, especially when not properly processed, also contain a high level of digestive inhibitors, known as anti-nutrients[39]. These inhibitors prevent the absorption of certain trace minerals like calcium and magnesium. They're known for their high protein content, but when examined against their carbohydrate content, the protein pales in comparison. For best results, don't consume legumes and this includes peanuts. Sorry peanut butter fans.

Alcohol consumption may be one of the leading causes of death and disease, directly or indirectly, in the western world. It reduces testosterone and fertility in men. It causes gut bacterial overgrowth, blood sugar issues, neurodegenerative diseases and a whole host of other consequences of inflammation[42]. Smoking is even worse for your health, and will prevent you from becoming an optimally functioning human being. At 21 years old, I put a halt to drinking alcohol to improve my health. You can too. These can be major addictions, so seek help if needed.

Soft drink and energy drink consumption are one of the quickest ways to earn yourself diabetes. It's also been shown to increase your risk for cancer, cardiovascular disease, Alzheimer's disease, and stroke among many other life-threatening conditions[43]. Feed your children this at your own will, but next time they can't concentrate at school or throw a tantrum in a public space, smack yourself on the arse for being such an idiot to give them a bottle of brain damage.

Keeping the theme of sugar rolling, fruit and especially fruit juice has become an onslaught to your liver, pancreas and your body's insulin receptors. Now I believe that some fruits are beneficial to include in the human diet, such as berries, papaya and pineapples (just not during the *Fresh Start*). But fruit, and in particular bananas, oranges and apples have been grown over the last century with one thing in mind - profit. These foods have been tampered with to produce plant-based lollies that are devoid of most of its once life-enhancing energy.

Fruit juice, especially the ones you don't make yourself, are so high in sugar that your body has no idea what to do with it. High fructose consumption, especially without the plant fibres, has been shown to increase very low-density lipoprotein (VLDL) particles, plus elevated insulin and triglycerides in the blood[44]. This means cardiovascular disease and diabetes. For lean, very active people, some fruits, like dates or prunes, consumed after training can aid in recovery and muscle growth, but for most men, you're better without.

Tea or Coffee?

Saving the best for last, let's talk about coffee. Known for its caffeine content, coffee increases levels of cortisol and adrenalin in the blood. These hormones have a stimulating effect on the body and activate the sympathetic nervous system. As I've mentioned before, one of the roles of cortisol is to break down muscle tissue and increase blood glucose. Here alone, we have two undesirable consequences: the loss of precious amino acids and a spike in blood sugar. When consumed regularly, chronic sympathetic nervous system stimulation may lead to anxiety, poor digestion, and even cognitive decline. Your brain adapts to the stimulant effects of coffee so from one per day, all of a sudden you need two, three, four and so on. One of my closest clients was drinking 40-50 long blacks per day during a particularly stressful period. Not surprisingly, this person suffered from terrible anxiety at this point in their life.

In today's high-pressure culture, coffee becomes a replacement for food. Just because you have energy doesn't mean you are nourished. By replacing food with coffee, you are depleting your body of vital nutrients like the amino acids glycine and glutamine, which are essential for a healthy brain and digestive system. Let's not forget that coffee is also causing extensive deforestation all over the planet, only to be thrown into landfill. In Australia, around one billion disposable, non-recyclable cups end up in landfill each year and take 20 years to decompose[45]. Most cups of coffee contain an unhealthy amount of agricultural chemicals, which may cause allergies, food intolerances and estrogenic effects in men[46].

For the majority of your life, you should stick with herbal tea. The world of tea is growing fast as the tremendous healing benefits of tea are being continuously discovered. Most teas are rich in antioxidants and phytonutrients, which prevent diseases, burn fat, and improve mental performance[47]. I've found that simply holding something warm in your hands mimics the feeling of holding your palms in front of a fire and creates a surge of feel-good chemicals, ultimately dampening cortisol.

If you enjoy your caffeine-hit too much to give up coffee, try a period of using green tea from Asia, yerba mate from South America, or the yaupon plant from North America. It may take some time to appreciate the new tastes, but it's worth it. These plants contain slightly less caffeine than coffee but have the added benefits of polyphenolic compounds like theanine and quercetin (antioxidants). When necessary, I prefer to use caffeine as a performance enhancing drug, and only when I am well-rested and well-fed. For all other times, it's delicious herbal blends.

This section wouldn't be complete without a note on product quality. While the jury is still out on the debate between organic food versus non-organic food, it's clear that local produce is a priority. Buying local means your food miles are low, which is good for the environment, and it also means more money in the farmer's pocket, which is right for the economy. Local food is always in season and will be fresher, tastier and more nutritious than those apples stored in cool rooms for eight months of the year. Grass-fed, pasture-raised, free-range animal products are essential here. As I have mentioned before, the healthier the animal is, the healthier you become.

What does all this look like?

Heeding these recommendations for a minimum of four weeks will be a challenge for most of you, but it will undoubtedly be worth it. You may be asking "What's left to eat?". I'll keep it simple: Meat, fats, and vegetables. See the below table for an example of a day in the life of an 80 kg male.

	Meal 1	**Meal 2**	**Meal 3**	**Meal 4**
Protein	Palm size Red Meat	Palm size Red Meat	Palm size White Meat	Palm size Fish
Fats	Thumb size Butter	Handful Macadamia Nuts	2 tbsp Olive Oil	1 Medium Avocado
Veg	Unlimited Green Veg	Unlimited Green Veg	Large bowl salad greens	Large plate roast veg
Other	Curry spices, Apple cider vinegar, Salt & pepper	Curry spices, Apple cider vinegar, Salt & pepper	Lemon, Fresh Herbs, Salt & Pepper	Lemon, Fresh Herbs, Salt & Pepper

As you can see from the plan above, I have included plenty of meat, fat, and salt. The perfect recipe for cardiovascular disease, right? In short, no. Fat is a primary component of our body. From sex hormones and cell membranes, to the physical structure of our brain, fat is an integral part of our biochemical makeup. There are no cultures on earth that successfully consume a low fat or low protein diet[37]. Conversely, it's entirely possible to consume low amounts of carbohydrates and function optimally.

In our society, it's very unnatural to have two tablespoons of butter melted into your meal, and this may take some adjustment. In traditional cultures, the throw away cuts of meat would be the lean muscle, while the head, tail and organs would be the most nutrient dense and first to be consumed[37]. The real culprit is vegetable oils, which are not usually made from vegetables but rather seeds. These contain a high amount of polyunsaturated fats that can be easily oxidised and cause free radical damage to your cells. If you eat more of the healthy fats like monounsaturated and saturated fat, then I guarantee, like many of my clients and myself, you will have more energy, focus and concentration as well as certain desire-enhancing effects.

An excellent quality salt, like Himalayan pink salt or Aztecan lake salt, can support so many functions of our body. From our nervous system to our adrenal glands, salt plays a critical role in keeping us alive. To prevent burnout or adrenal fatigue, the best solution is salt. One of my female clients was working in a high-stress position, looking after two children by herself and managing a tumultuous relationship with her husband. She was suffering severe adrenal fatigue, and all she wanted to do was drink salt, vinegar and oil. People were telling her she was crazy. I told her that she was intuitive.

I have seen high cholesterol in people that consume a low fat, low salt diet. These people are incredibly stressed, and their body reacts to this stress by pumping more cholesterol carrying proteins into the blood. I ask them to reduce their stress and increase their salt and fat intake, and they sleep better, have more energy, lose body fat, and their blood markers improve out of sight.

Some signs and symptoms to look out for salt deficiency are insomnia, tinnitus, vertigo and even facial muscle spasms or paralysis. Adrenal fatigue is a serious problem and must be addressed as soon as possible. Just to be extremely clear, most people living and working in a city have some degree of adrenal stress.

It's has been shown that the biggest contributors to cardiovascular disease are sugar consumption and stress[48]. These cause damage to your blood vessels, promoting plaque formation, which leads to an increased risk of cardiovascular disease. Deliciously, the French were right all along. So relax, and consume your salty, fatty foods, providing that they come from organic, grass-fed/wild-caught sources and are not highly processed packaged foods.

Gut health is also a factor in contributing not just to cardiovascular disease, but autoimmune conditions and cognitive decline[41]. The bacteria within us play an incredibly diverse role in our physiology, and this must not be overlooked. Any changes to diet and lifestyle affect our gut bacteria, and the adoption of the *Fresh Start* will only have positive results for your intestinal health.

Initially, clients often complain about the challenge of eating four meals each day. This struggle is due to the hormonal cascade that occurs throughout our busy day. When we are stressed, we suppress our hunger hormones, because finding food isn't a priority when that lion is chasing you. If we go too long without food, we crave sweets, coffee or other foods that stimulate the reward systems of the brain. If this occurs, your engine is running off sugar, which we now understand to be completely unsustainable.

It's imperative to prioritise regular eating to mitigate these physiological stress responses. It should be obvious that famine is an added stressor that your body may not tolerate well, especially over prolonged periods - as in the case with fanatical fasting practitioners. So, in the beginning, I encourage you to eat four meals each day and regulate your energy intake through the amount of food in each meal.

My father had a chronic shoulder injury that according to the doctor and physiotherapist, required surgery. He tried to eliminate this chronic pain through yoga and physical therapy but to no avail. He eventually had the surgery, but found that even after six months, he wasn't feeling any better. He was taking anti-inflammatory drugs and avoiding excessive movement. Nothing was helping. Luckily his son is an evangelical health nut, and eventually persuaded him to undertake the *Fresh Start*. Two weeks later the shoulder pain was barely noticeable. We both cheered with victory.

During a conversation a few weeks later, I checked back in with his injury.

"How's the shoulder?", I said.

"Meh, it's back to how it was", Dad replied.

"How are you eating at the moment?", I rebutted.

His voice changed, "Um like I was before I guess, bread and sweets have crept back in, and I'm drinking wine again", he murmured.

With a sense of arrogance but also frustration, I replied. "I rest my case".

Never underestimate the power that food has on your body. From chronic pain, to debilitating diseases, it may be a simple switch of nutrition that has the profound, fountain-of-youth effect you have long been seeking. It's time to experiment. Clean out your kitchen and start cooking with real foods.

Chapter Eleven

Nutrients In, Scales Out

"Health is not about the weight you lose, but about the life you gain!".

- Dr Josh Axe

Among any counter-culture philosophy - such as the atypical advice found in this book - there is a message that goes against the general dogma so deeply that it makes some people's brains melt. It causes a great divide among the people, with deeply entrenched conservatives on one side and radical progressives on the other.

The same is true in nutrition, and the message is this: "Calories in versus calories out". Otherwise stated, "Your body, with its millions of internal biochemical processes, is as simple as a steam engine. When you put fuel into the engine, it must burn, or it gets fat". Forget hormones such as adiponectin, leptin, growth hormone, testosterone, DHEA and progesterone. Never mind considering fuel sources such as lactate, glucose and ketones. And don't worry about essential nutrients such as zinc, magnesium, glycine and EPA. Fuel is fuel, and the amount of energy you put in is the amount of energy you get out.

Obviously, I am hypercritical of mainstream conversation, but in 2017, there are still hundreds of thousands of health practitioners around the world that believe this oversimplified message of health. Thankfully, for your appetite and taste buds,

I'm here to tell you that this is completely and utterly wrong.

The problem with this belief is that the message does not include a discussion of nutrient density. "If it fits your macros" is touted by the bodybuilders (as they chow down on a litre of Ben and Jerry's on their cheat day), but in my view, this is total neglect of your body. How is 1000 calories of pizza equal to 1000 calories of slow-cooked wallaby shank with vegetables?

It's not. For example, let's take two different breakfasts. One is had by millions of Australians every day: Vegemite on toast. The other, I believe is much more Australian and eat most mornings: Kangaroo mince & vegetable curry.

If we took 500 calories of these two meals, we would see a vastly different nutrient profile across the board. From crucial amino acids to essential minerals, it would surprise me to see Vegemite on toast outperform a kanga curry in any nutrient. Not only would we see an increase in nutrients for my breakfast but there are also less toxic food materials such as gluten, sugar, pesticides and preservatives. It is ridiculous to compare foods purely for their caloric content.

Nowhere was this advice more apparent than while coaching at 5EW. Every new member would be instructed to eat according to the *Fresh Start* of the previous chapter and under no circumstances should portion control be implemented. In fact, I often recommended that people eat as much as they possibly can.

This is because the typical situation for a person when beginning a health journey is that they have been unconsciously starving themselves for so long, sometimes many decades. The mainstream dogma of not overeating is so ingrained in our psyche that even the biggest men had been under-eating for most of their adult life. This led their bodies to a state of chronic starvation and hormonal resistance, particularly of the hormones leptin, adrenaline and insulin, which are all essential for burning fat.

Not only does not eating enough food long term cause you to store more body fat, but it also ages you incredibly fast. Have you ever noticed how when grandma loses her appetite, she grows frail and demented unbelievably quick? It would be revolutionary if nursing homes fed their community a diet of bone broths, animal fats and fermented vegetables rather than a sugar-laden diet of commercial yoghurt and toast. Incredibly, our brain is made up of mostly fat and craves it as a fuel source.

As I began doing monthly assessments for members of 5EW, it was beautiful to see the benefits of removing portion control and allowing unlimited healthy foods onto the plate and into the belly. Particularly for men, who have a much more durable metabolism than women, it was easy to recommend that they eat more of these foods and watch the fat drop off, their skin grow tighter, their face looks younger, and they report of unbelievably stable energy throughout their day's work.

This is partly because they are flooding their body with nutrients like zinc, selenium and vitamin E and partly because they are rebalancing hormonal ratios that are essential for youth such as DHEA and cortisol. When our bodies become stressed, such as during a period of famine, cortisol is elevated, and DHEA is suppressed. DHEA is important for muscle mass, fat distribution, sexual desire and energy production among many other things. It is made of pregnenolone, which comes from cholesterol and vitamin B6, two very essential nutrients that are not found in our typical Aussie breakfast.

The reason that cortisol elevates during periods of famine is that its role is to break down proteins from muscle, bones and your organs into amino acids. It then converts these amino acids into glucose so that your brain has some instant energy and does not shut off. Thank you cortisol, maybe you're not *all* bad.

The unfortunate thing is that when we overuse cortisol, like during stressful days at work or excessive coffee consumption, we chronically break down our body's protein stores and raise our blood glucose levels. This is how not eating enough food, when combined with eating the wrong foods, can eventually lead to type 2 diabetes.

Even when I first joined the team at 5EW, I thought I was eating a high amount of healthy calories, mainly from fats. It turns out, upon calculation, I was supplying my body with only around 1,800 calories every day. For the amount of work and training that I was aspiring to do, my body required almost double that, a total of 3,500 calories. As soon as I switched my mindset from "I'll eat just enough to get through the day" to "I'll eat as much as I possibly can", my energy went through the roof, my libido returned and my consistent allergic reactions completely disappeared.

My favourite example is a close friend and 5EW member named Mark. Mark is 51 and has been physically active his entire life. He is a plumber by trade and has owned a successful building business for 30 years. This man has more life-force running through him than almost anyone I've ever met. Over his time at 5EW, Mark built his caloric intake to 4,400 calories per day. Over this same period, he dropped 6.5% body fat.

Furthermore, when Mark reduced his food intake during some experiments in intermittent fasting, he put on body fat. It was clear that Mark was running at such high revolutions per minute that his body demanded more nutrients. When he ate more food, his hormones functioned better, and he felt unstoppable. Eating four and a half thousand calories per day is not easy, nor cheap, but Mark enjoys a six-pack in all seasons of the year and could take on almost any man half his age.

When you are on your journey of health and fitness, it is especially important not to look at the scales. The reason for this is that it is very likely you will put on muscle, particularly if you are doing strength training. Muscle weighs much more than fat by volume and so even if you weigh the same, your clothes will fit a lot more loosely if your body fat percentage is reduced by 10%.

Watching the scales move day-by-day can be very discouraging; the best form of body composition measurement in my view, for simplicity and expense is the camera. There are more accurate, data-driven and expensive forms of analysis available, but in my opinion, a simple photograph tells a thousand words. You will easily know when you have dropped body fat and built muscle.

If you don't care for body image and are reading this book just to better your health, then more power to you. Once I found my ideal body shape, I haven't taken a photo nor skinfold measurement in years, and I believe I am happier for it. If you've read up to this point, you probably agree that body fat measurement is a means to an end, not the end itself.

If you are to be successful in health as a man who carries a lot of responsibilities in your daily life, you need to eat accordingly. Consume 4 to 5 meals of nutrient dense food every day. If you believe that you may be eating too much food, it's much healthier to move your body more rather than to starve yourself. You have put your body through enough famine. It's time to ditch portion control and feast.

Chapter Twelve

The Art of Supplementation

"Nothing should be done without a purpose".

- Marcus Aurelius

Flash back to the Travers' family kitchen, late 2011. My brother is staring at me in pure disgust. In my hands, I held a concoction of super foods so vile that the pungent smell was causing him to dry-retch. In this brew was algae, wild roots, and exotic fruits from all over the planet stirred into 250 ml of water. It was supposed to make me virile and strong-like-bull. Man, was I healthy? Right? ...Guys?

From rhino horns, to tiger penis, to Modafinil, and steroids, the world has always been obsessed with something that will make us bigger, stronger, faster, and smarter. Or, at the least, aid the male ego. We want to outsource as much hard work as possible to a magic pill or potion that will do the job for us. Whether it's improving libido, building muscle, burning fat or boosting IQ, there is *surely* some combination out there that will make us feel like we're Bradley Cooper on the movie Limitless.

Unfortunately, more often than not, any given new drug is usually just a great way for the manufacturer to make a tonne of money. Sometimes the supplement you take has little to no effect, and sometimes it's outright dangerous. It's time to clear the fog and see which supplements you actually may need to consume, and which you can throw out of your musty medicine cabinet.

In my short life, I have spent tens of thousands of dollars on supplements from alpha-lipoic acid to zinc and everything in between. At one point, my morning smoothie probably cost more than a fancy restaurant breakfast, despite being much less palatable. When I arrived at 5EW, I learned that I was very likely over supplementing to the point of potential damage to my liver and digestive system. I was doing this because I didn't have my own well thought out supplementation system. I was broken and needed help, but I didn't know what to do. After my 12-week 5EW *Leaky Gut Protocol*, I understood that there was a process to supplementation. In fact, it's more of an art; a gut feeling, you could say.

Thankfully, I learnt the process of reviewing our client's blood panels. Our onsite doctor measured over 50 different blood markers, from a full blood count, to levels of essential vitamins and minerals; we were fortunate to have this kind of insight to then prescribe supplementation, nutritional outlines, exercise programmes and lifestyle habits.

I rarely recommended more than five supplements for someone to take at any one period. I always preferred to try to solve the issue with food or a new lifestyle habit. These five supplements came from a larger group of about eight. While we had dozens of supplements at the facility, I rarely used most of them with my clients unless they presented with a complex issue.

Let's talk about my eight most commonly prescribed supplements.

Responsible for nearly 300 enzymatic processes in the body, healthy zinc levels are a foundation of exceptional men's health. It is most readily obtained in high amounts in oysters, red meat and pumpkin seeds. The functions of zinc are almost endless, but among them are to enhance immune cell function, increase free testosterone, balance blood sugar levels, increase serotonin and reduce inflammation. It is very effective at reducing symptoms of chronic inflammatory conditions such as rheumatoid arthritis. Some symptoms of low zinc can be fatigue, depression, digestive issues, brittle hair and nails, loss of appetite and acne. It's also the most efficient mineral to reduce gynecomastia, AKA the dreaded man-boobs. Depending on your symptoms, blood levels and body weight I recommend between 60-150 mg/day with breakfast.

Almost everyone that I have worked with says that this magic mineral is their favourite supplement. The fourth most abundant mineral in your body, magnesium is the closest thing to the fountain of youth, because it has a calming effect on the nervous system and directly reduces chronic cortisol levels. Supplementation reduces cortisol by actually boosting the hormone di-dehydroepiandrosterone or DHEA[49], which is converted into the anabolic hormone, testosterone. Magnesium promotes learning and memory as a result of its beneficial effect on synaptic plasticity and density[50]. Much like zinc, magnesium is responsible for hundreds of different processes in the body which include reducing stress, improving sleep, heart health, increasing bone density, regulating blood sugar, liver detoxification, as well as a positive effect on mood via dopamine[50]. Symptoms of low magnesium can be wide-ranging, from low libido and poor sleep patterns, to high blood pressure and headaches. Ideally you should take 10 mg/kg of body weight (800 mg for an 80 kg male), half at 4 p.m., half at 7 p.m. By supplementing with magnesium, you're helping to protect yourself against deadly diseases and significantly improve the quality of your life.

Slip, slop, slap was the slogan that struck fear into my heart as a child. The sun was the enemy, and I was to dodge it from umbrella to umbrella for the rest of my life. This rhetoric has caused vitamin D deficiency for so many Australians. Vitamin D regulates about five percent of your entire genome. That's about 4,000 different genetic expressions that can be turned on or off with vitamin D. From autoimmunity to cancer, vitamin D plays a vital role in preventing diseases. For me, our society's chronic vitamin D deficiency is a sign that our lifestyle is so far removed from our original hunter-gatherer way of living and that we are not living following our biology. Supplementing this should only be based on blood panel results, as high levels can be toxic and cause calcium accumulation in tissues. As mentioned earlier however, a pill can never replace being in nature and under the sun.

Essential for thousands of different functions, the B vitamin group are always saddening for me to prescribe. It should be straightforward to get enough B vitamins from your food, but frankly, most people don't eat the right foods, let alone eat enough food at all. I've never seen a vegan or vegetarian with adequate levels of B12 without supplementation, and this can sometimes explain any neurological conditions that long-term vegetarians may experience. Symptoms of deficiencies are so vast that it could be impossible to diagnose effectively. It's best to get your blood levels tested and supplement accordingly. Foods highest in B vitamins are herring, sardines, red meat and offal.

If you manage to get blood readings of the above nutrients, it's preferable to be on the mid-upper end of the therapeutic range.

Fish oil is one of the most widely researched supplements on the planet. Study after study shows that a supplement containing high amounts of DHA and EPA helps reduce inflammation and improve blood glucose management. In my own experience, high dose cod liver oil was one of the main components that helped me eliminate the allergic reaction from my skin. There is some debate about the effectiveness of omega-3 supplements due to the fact that they are indeed polyunsaturated fatty acids, which are the most unstable fatty acid. However, I have found that they are incredibly effective at helping to reduce inflammation and improve blood glucose management in the early stages of one's health journey. Once you are 12 to 24 months into eating a paleo-style diet, long-term supplementation will likely become unnecessary. Liquid forms are almost always better than capsules, and it's best to get your source from small, cold-water fish like arctic cod-liver oil. Taking 5-10 ml per day is perfect for maintenance.

It's been said that all disease begins in the gut. I can testify that chronic gut inflammation is indeed a huge cause, or at least, major contributor to not only debilitating conditions like irritable bowel disease or Crohn's, but also to skin problems, mental health disorders, allergies, chronic joint pain, frequent colds and flus, obesity and much more. There are entire books written on the human micro-biome as we continue to discover the incredibly vital role that our gut bacteria play in our physiology. From preventing autoimmune conditions and learning disabilities to your preference of food and even your sexual partner, these little bugs inside your digestive tract are controlling your thoughts and actions more than you realise.

I have the unique privilege of reviewing clients stool test results and often see very little to no healthy beneficial bacteria in the gut. If this is the case, I recommend a four week course of 450 billion bacteria per day for 30-days. Vivomixx or VSL#3 are the most well-known products. An appropriate maintenance dose would be 50-100 billion bacteria, consisting of Lactobacillus species, Bifidobacterium species, Bacillus species, Streptococcus thermophilus and often times even Escherichia coli.

Unfortunately, our stressed and sterile lifestyle is creating a desert wasteland inside our intestines, and this leaves us open for anything to take residences, such as nasty candida or toxic gram-negative bacteria. Toxins such as lipopolysaccharides and acetaldehyde are released and can overload the liver and immune system leading to intestinal permeability, allergies, and cognitive decline[51]. The detrimental effects of these inhabitants can be catastrophic and should be dealt with by an expert in treating gut dysfunction. Inquire at a holistic doctor or skilled naturopath if they perform comprehensive digestive stool analysis. Regarding these tests, you get what you pay for, so be prepared to fork out a few hundred dollars for the test itself. I repeat, the journey to remove these nasties successfully should not be undergone alone.

One safe, food-based supplement that is helpful to every client and their guts is apple cider vinegar (ACV). This potent tonic tastes absolutely vile to most initiates but, over a few weeks of regular consumption, begins to emanate the sweetness of apples. Start with one teaspoon of organic ACV in one litre of water, sipping throughout the day, and eventually increase to one tablespoon per litre. Your whole body, from your belly to your skin, will thank you for it.

Glutamine is a conditionally-essential amino acid, meaning it can mostly be made by the body except under situations of stress or pathology. Unfortunately, these stressful conditions are much more common than they should be. During my *Leaky Gut Protocol*, I consumed 80 g or four tablespoons of glutamine in water each day for four weeks. Glutamine is one of the amino acids that converts readily into glucose with the help of cortisol, so supplementing it can have a muscle sparing effect. For maintenance, most practitioners recommend 5-10 g after strength training, but in my experience, this dose is negligible and should be increased to 20-40 g. Glutamine is helpful in the production of secretory IgA, a defensive immunoglobulin located in your gut. It also helps the epithelial cells of your intestinal lining digest and absorbs your food. Finally, it's involved in the production of glutathione, arguably your most important antioxidant.

Protein shakes, and other amino acids should only be used for individuals with extremely high training volume and therefore a lot of food consumption. It is much more effective to get these nutrients from food, as the cofactors and other nutrients that come from food benefit your body in ways that we haven't even discovered. So if your full-time job isn't eating to gain mass, then these supplements are likely not worth your time or money. If you're consuming protein shakes, make sure they are organic, with no fillers, preservatives, colours, or flavours.

If the above recommendations are overwhelming and you're after a simpler method of supplementation, then simply avoid products containing any of the following:

1. An insanely ripped man wearing sunglasses (either animated or real) on the front.
2. Promises of enough energy to wrestle a gorilla.
3. More ingredients than a Christmas Lunch.
4. Names ending in "Max", "Pro", or any multiple of 1000.

There are many blog articles out there claiming to know the best practices for supplementation. The unfortunate thing is that most of these articles are selling their own products. My only intention is to educate you on this complex topic; by investigating platforms such as Examine.com and LabDoor you can do your further research.

I'm thankful that I have come a long way from taking dangerous pre-workout formulas such as SuperPump-250 and Jack3D all those years ago. The promise of a dramatic boost in manliness was too much for a naive young boy to pass up. With the information above you can now navigate the murky waters of the supplement industry with more clarity and direction.

Chapter Thirteen

What's Good for You is Good for Them

"From a small seed a mighty trunk may grow".

- *Aeschylus*

I strode in to greet my regular Friday 6 p.m. client who was warming up on the rowing machine. "How are you?", I said. He was quite gleeful this evening; he replied that he was fantastic, and super excited to take his sons to a notorious pancake restaurant for dinner. My heart sank.

Looking to understand why he felt this was alright, I reminded him that he had been working with me for nearly 18 months; exercising, experiencing the benefits of nutrition, cultivating a new lifestyle, and developing healthy habits. He was setting such a great example for his kids at home, and they were proud.

He said to me, almost asking for forgiveness, "But Jordy, they're just kids".

With a smile, I rebutted, "If they're just kids, why are they eating the 'food' that will cause them to end up in the same position you were, whilst you get to eat only the best nutrition available? If all you want is a good sleep, a stable mood, steady energy and the ability to fight of disease, don't your kids deserve to have that same level of health? Think about what good nutrition means to you, it means the same to them, especially because they're kids. We can't forget that they have a human body that is fueled in just the same way as ours. They just have more potential".

He looked off into the distance for a few moments, quietly weighing up the consequences of a pancake-less evening, then turned back to me and said, "You're right".

It definitely struck a pain point for me discussing this with my client. My own parents, like most, did their best with the knowledge they had at the time. Evidence for the connection between a child's nutrition and physical or psychological dysfunction is becoming more and more apparent. With the vastly different knowledge we have now, one can't help but consider the potential of lives fueled properly, and also the cost to those who miss out. The knowledge we have now can potentially save a child (who will be an adult hopefully 90% of their life) from chronic illnesses, disabilities, mental disorders and even sporting injuries. We are so incredibly fortunate to have this evidence now at our fingertips. We mustn't ignore the evidence, especially because 'they're just kids'.

One of the most common problems that children suffer is an inability to manage blood glucose levels. The typical child is tortured with a wild see-saw between hyperglycemia (high blood sugar) and hypoglycemia (low blood sugar) all throughout the day. Dr. Campbell-McBride reports in her book *Gut and Psychology Syndrome*, "It has been proven that a lot of hyperactivity, inability to concentrate and learn, aggression and other behavioral abnormalities in school children are a direct result of this glucose roller coaster. The hyperglycemic phase produces a feeling of a "high" with hyperactive, manic tendencies… While the hypoglycemic phase makes them feel unwell, often with a headache, bad mood, tantrums, aggression and general fatigue…"[52].

Taking the same approach for us adults, I believe a lot of marital arguments may be prevented by the simple act of having some food. When our blood sugar drops, we become irritable and frustrated quickly, and this can lead to unreasonable and unnecessary (hangry) quarrels. But it's not just about having some food to stabilise our blood sugar, it's also about what food we ate, three to five hours earlier. Was it strawberry jam on toast, or a slow-cooked lamb shoulder with vegetables? And yes, the latter option is breakfast meal guaranteed to set you up for a successful day - don't let the cereal companies convince you otherwise.

Another leading cause of disease and dysfunction in children is the inflammatory conditions that arise from out-of-control intestinal bacteria[50.] Overgrowth of specific bacteria such as Candida species and Clostridia species have been linked with autism, A.D.H.D, schizophrenia, and depression[50,53]. These bacterial complications stem as early in the child's life as birth. Dr. David Perlmutter shows in his book *Brain Maker* that there is evidence that newborns from cesarean births are deprived of life-enhancing bacteria that arise from the mother's vagina, and are much more likely to develop digestive issues and neurological dysfunction later in life[51]. It's also likely that an unhealthy mother gives birth to a sick baby, even if the birth was natural. It's with this understanding that we realise our health not only impacts ourselves but our closest loved ones too.

To alleviate digestive dysfunction, we must heal the intestinal microbiome and also the gut lining. The best-known method is through diet. Foods high in fat and protein and low in carbohydrates (particularly starch), have been shown to improve digestive disorders and also neurological symptoms in children[50]. It's important to recognise that children can often tolerate more carbohydrates than adults, so this low carbohydrate approach should only be used with children suffering digestive or neurological dysfunction.

A much safer blanket approach is to remove all processed foods including bread, pasta, sugar, dairy, soy, and especially anything containing artificial colours and flavours. As early as 1975, a study showed "a rapid improvement in behaviour and learning abilities in ADHD children following dietary management eliminating artificial food colours, flavours, and naturally occurring salicylates[54]". These foods cause a myriad of problems concerning the human body from neurological and DNA damage to chronic inflammation[50].

Another family that I work with only consumes foods from organic health food stores and local farmer's markets. On one exceptional occasion, they needed to visit a supermarket chain. Whilst cruising down an aisle, their eight-year-old boy exclaimed, "Mum! This is it!".

"This is what, honey?", His mum replied.

Wide eyed, he responded, "THIS is where my friends get all that stuff from!".

The two were in the confectionary aisle, and this school boy had never seen the items in their packaging on the shelves, let alone in his own pantry. His parents and I are open and honest about their child rearing experiences. They've never had complaints about poor mood or hyperactivity, he's never been out of control, or struggling to learn in school. If you're questioning whether theirs is a healthy approach to parenting, I would invite you to challenge your own approach.

Returning to the pancake story, the real issue was that the father honestly just didn't realise the implications of what his children were eating. Even though his middle son had learning disabilities, and he often complained to me that all three were playing up, he didn't connect the dots on his own. When you've been misinformed all your life, you almost can't blame him.

To better regulate your family's blood sugar levels, intestinal microbiome, and overall health, you must apply the same rules as we discussed earlier. What's healthy for you is healthy for them. Yes, there can be some variances in genetics and physiology depending on the phase of one's life. But for the most part, if you remove processed foods and takeaway meals, and instead cook and prepare your food together, not only are you ensuring your child's success in sport and school (and therefore life), but you are also teaching them vital food-specific skills and knowledge for them to teach the next generation.

Chef Pete Evans is spearheading the healthy food in schools crusade in Australia that Jamie Oliver so successfully kick-started throughout the UK. Pete says it best in his blog: "Variety is the spice of life, so I encourage you to continue to be bold and brave with the foods you introduce your kids too. By encouraging adventurous palettes, you'll ensure they have a lifelong love affair with what they put in their mouths, and their physical and emotional health can benefit tremendously. Ultimately, as a parent, it's all about trusting that the invaluable food knowledge you give your kids will pay off when they are on their own and that they will be well equipped to easily make the right choices"[55]. Understanding and delighting in food as medicine is indeed an empowering prospect that will serve us all now and for generations to come.

Changing your perspective on your family's nutrition is a cornerstone on which to build your investment in lifelong health and happiness. With your loved ones, I also invite you to explore the other tricks and tips throughout this book, and have fun with it. From meditation and breathing, to cold showers and movement, experience these with your children or your loving partner. Learning and exploring together will strengthen your relationships. Watching one another flourish is the ultimate reward.

Part Three: Nutrition - Summary

Remember that there is no one perfect diet that everybody can eat.

1. Your optimal nutrition is unique to your body.

Complete the *Fresh Start*.

2. Commit to four weeks of eliminating the following foods:
    Grains
    Gluten
    Dairy
    Soy
    Sugar and soft drink
    Artificial colours or flavours
    Coffee
    Alcohol
    Fruit and fruit juice
    Legumes

Forget starving yourself.

3. Focus on consuming as many nutrients as you can.
4. Eat four meals each day.

Use supplements intelligently.

5. Stick to the big three:
    1. Magnesium for detoxification, sleep and stress management.
        10mg/kg bodyweight (800mg for an 80kg person) every evening.
    2. Zinc for testosterone, immunity and skin health.
        60-150mg daily with breakfast.
    3. Fish oil for reducing inflammation and improving blood sugar management.
        5-10ml daily

Encourage your family to join you on your health journey.

6. Don't accept the normal standards for children's nutrition.

7. Change is much easier when all parties are committed.

movement

Chapter Fourteen

Because You're Human

"Without movement, life is unthinkable".

- Moshé Feldenkrais

"Movement equals life". These were some of the first words uttered to me by one of my mentors. "No movement, no life!". I was in Sydney's Bondi district in an intimate group of students, learning from arguably the world's best movement teacher, philosopher, artist and practitioner, Ido Portal. I knew I was in for a life-changing week.

His most profound lessons did not come through biomechanical analysis of complex movements. That wasn't Ido's concern. His focus was on delivering a new way to look at human movement differently, which is to say he shows you how to look at human life differently. If there's not enough movement in your life, you will decay. If there is too much movement, which is in the case of professional athletes and performers, you will experience injury and bodily breakdown. The people that I commonly work with suffer from a movement deficiency. As a result, their body decays, they develop pains, aches, weaknesses and immobility. This is not sustainable nor respectful for the only body that you have been given.

For Ido, and now myself, a movement practice is the same as a life practice. How you prioritise movement is how much you prioritise life. The level of movement you incorporate into your weekly calendar could reflect the level of integrity you have to your humanness. One of the best ways to develop new neural networks is through movement. Portal said, "The brain is intended for movement complexity, and likely not technological advancements. Movement complexity is one of the reasons that we have evolved. We can move in more complex ways than any other animal. Consider that no animal can mimic us better than we can mimic it". This ability helped us to hunt, communicate at long distance and even develop unique cultural practices like singing, storytelling, and dancing.

To move in complex ways is a part of our genetic makeup. If we do not use this ability, we can see a breaking down of the body, from neurodegenerative diseases to arthritis. Movement complexity is greater than simple movements repeated over and over. For example, a rock climber will be a much better movement practitioner than someone who practices chin-ups for the sake of fitness. A martial artist, who reacts to their environment, will be more masterful than a yogi, who is confined to their mat. It's up to you to explore the universe of movement as much as you can. Your humanness will thank you.

It sounds rather unsettling, but remember, we evolved over hundreds of thousands of years, interacting with nature, swinging from trees, climbing rocks and swimming. Today however, we're far removed from our natural human environment. We now sit in a chair, hunched over a desk, under artificial light, breathing stale air, wearing restrictive clothing and experiencing a cascade of stress hormones. Our food is grown, harvested, processed and packaged for us, often hundreds of kilometres away. Our need to walk hundreds of kilometres each week is outsourced to motor-vehicles and other transport. The human race continues to evolve according to the stimulus we give our genetic material. There is no pause button on evolution.

Biomechanist, Katy Bowman developed a concept which she

calls movement ecology. This illustrates the effect that our environment has on our movement patterns as well as the effect that our movement patterns have on the environment. When one goes to forage, for example, the act of trampling over shrubbery and pulling leaves and berries off of a bush stimulates new growth within the environment. Conversely, when you are stuck in a concrete jungle, the environment forces you to conform. Your sleek leather shoes mould your toes together, your chair binds your hips, and the noise of the busy streets forces your hearing to become less sensitive.

Bowman even suggests that the chronic underuse of our full length of vision is a contributing cause to the epidemic of short-sightedness. For the majority of our waking hours, we use less than 0.5% of our maximum distance of vision. When we look up from our smartphone or computer, we can often only stare as far as the wall. If we want to preserve our vision, it is imperative we give our eyes something to focus on far off in the distance. This is not movement as we typically think of it, but this information is just as critical for the preservation of our species.

In her book, *Movement Matters*, Bowman illustrates movement ecology with a simple image of a glorious orca with it's fin flopped over. No orca has ever been seen in the wild with a flaccid fin. This led activists against Sea World to believe that the orca was protesting it's capture by flopping it's fin to one side. After some research, marine biologists revealed that the fin had flopped over because it was no longer being encouraged to stand tall by the immense pressures of deep-sea diving that the orca performed in the wild. We understand that this new environment was shaping the physical structure of the animal.

The same occurs in any animal, including you. If we zoom in on the physiological effects of sitting down all day, we not only see chronically tight hip flexors and weak pelvic muscles, we see an increased risk of cardiovascular disease. The reason for this may be due to the turbulence in blood flow that occurs through major blood vessels[31]. This can damage the cells and cause the need for plaque formation, which given the new damage to the blood vessel wall, would be an appropriate biological response, except it also increases the risk for cardiovascular disease.

A similar situation occurs when we eliminate our bowels. Sitting down on a toilet seat constricts the junction between the intestines and the rectum. This constriction naturally causes a blockage, leading to constipation and straining, and eventually nasty implications like haemorrhoids and even bowel cancer[31]. The alternative to sitting down is, well, squatting. When you squat the ligament that surrounds this area in your bowels releases, and you experience an easy removal of your biological waste.

What's a man to do? I mentioned this earlier, but it bears repeating: I give you the awesome team at Knees Up: The Healthy Stool: "The Knees Up lets you remain in a natural position, each and every time you poo. What's awesome about this is that when you squat instead of sit, you'll be able to fully eliminate all of your waste each and every time. Not only does squatting straighten your insides up and relaxes your puborectalis muscle, allowing for free flow, but it also completely empties your system without any strain. This prevents fecal stagnation and the accumulation of toxins in your intestinal tract".

I have used variations of squatting tools from a stack of books to the Squatty Potty and found each of them to be oh so smooth. For an unforgettable dose of toilet humour, watch the YouTube epic This Unicorn Changed the Way I Poop #SquattyPotty. Pimp out your alone time with this elegant device; it'll be the talk of the table at your next dinner party.

Bowman sums up movement ecology in one powerful

sentence: "In nature, there are no rewards or punishments, only consequences". It seems that the less we behave like our ancestors, the more deleterious our health becomes. Human movement is the best way to encourage ancestral behaviour and bring us back to a natural state of health.

Our society believes that spending three to four hours per week dedicated to movement is a healthy way to live. While working at 5EW, I discovered that my best results with clients came when they moved more often. The more often I saw someone moving, the more body fat they lost and the more energy they had. It became evident that the more movement they integrated into the day, the more lively they became.

Of course, there is a danger of over-training, but if the level of intensity and type of movement pattern is varied enough, you could move for many hours every day of the week. From fasted walking every morning to crawling on the floor like a lizard, the various ways in which you can move are vast. It simply requires you to be intelligent and creative about how you operate your body.

Science has discovered countless benefits to exercising, but I wonder how many advantages we will continue to uncover as time goes on. Consider the nature of the above movement, the lizard crawl. Your spine undulates with every step to conform with the floor. The muscles of your entire body develop strength in extreme, end-range positions. Your bones experience load in new ways and begin to lay down more minerals to become stronger. Your lungs expand and contract as you breathe to remove carbon dioxide. Your diaphragm works overtime, pumping the lymphatic fluid around your body, clearing waste and cellular debris. The driver of this body, your brain, tries to understand the most efficient way for you to move through space. Your heart pumps freshly oxygenated blood, delivering life to each cell. Your sebaceous glands secrete salty fluid to cool your overheating body. Your skin all over your body is stretched, massaged and stimulated in every way imaginable. You are covered in sweat. An intense surge of endorphins flood your body. You feel alive.

So how do you begin to revive your body? Start by moving more. Move every day in different ways, for as long as you can. As you feel comfortable with one practice, change it. The human body only evolves with learning and refining new movement patterns. As Portal would say, "Get good at what you don't do". It's not only incredibly boring, but it has little merit to be performing the same movements in the gym for decades on end. Continuously increase the level of complexity, in which your body moves through space. It may only take a few minutes to perfect the nature of a bicep curl, but to perfect the complex movements of a mixed martial artist may take an entire lifetime.

Chapter Fifteen

No Cardio, No Worries

"Research your own experience; absorb what is useful, reject what is useless and add what is essentially your own".

- *Bruce Lee*

What if I told you there was a way to lose body fat and feel unstoppable without spending ten hours on a bike saddle or pounding the pavement for dozens of kilometres each week? There's a growing number of middle aged men that are gravitating towards cycling, due to its low impact form of exercise, as well as the opportunity to grab a latte and muffin with your mates; but there is a much more efficient and healthier way to move your body. Enter strength training.

My boss, an ex-marathoner, often joked that there is no better way to turn a man into a woman than by forcing him to perform endurance training. Of course, he was facetious, however the damaging effects of excessive endurance training can be true, particularly for overworked and underfed men.

Endurance training raises cortisol for a constant and extended period. If you combine this with caffeine and the heinous act of skipping breakfast, then you're entering a catabolic state, categorised by a breakdown of lean muscle, which is converted to glucose; a process known as gluconeogenesis.

I have seen this with many of my clients. Matt, a 43-year-old long-time recreational cyclist, started working with me to get stronger for an international cycling trip in six months time. I encouraged him to stop cycling while we work to improve his biomechanical imbalances. Matt's entire upper body was incredibly tight, he had no glutes and was nowhere near being able to touch his toes.

We started training squats with just the weight of the bar alone, and learning how to activate the muscles of his posterior chain. He was eating according to the *Fresh Start* and then, after 4-weeks, began eating carbohydrates for extra fuel as he was already quite lean. In less than 12 weeks he lost 5.3% body fat, and added 2 kg of muscle. Matt had lost over 3 kg of body weight and was now the strongest he'd ever been in his entire life, which is incredibly important for a power-to-weight ratio sport like cycling.

Strength training is the act of improving strength, and often also the quality and size of our muscle. We achieve this by moving a joint under load, which can be either a barbell, atlas stone or your bodyweight. Powerlifting, Olympic weightlifting, strongman training and calisthenics all fall under the umbrella of strength training. When taught by a professional, it's safe and incredibly rewarding to make progress.

I was fortunate enough to learn various methods of strength training during my time at 5EW, and saw tremendous benefits to my physique, my energy levels, and my ability to function in everyday life. Carrying heavy or awkward objects was no longer a chore but a rewarding challenge. One of my clients, Andrew, enjoys boundless energy while playing with his eight-year-old boy after two years of strength training.

Powerlifting is often thought to be reserved for ape-like men who struggle to walk through doors, but it's the foundation we teach strength from. People need to learn how to deadlift a straight bar before they can pick up a heavy stone from the floor. To achieve the size and strength of the enormous men you have seen on TV, you would need to eat four to six times the amount of food you currently eat, and be in the gym for at least ten hours per week. So fear not, this is a safe practice to engage in.

Strongman training has occurred throughout the world over thousands of years. From lifting concrete stones in ancient Greece, to the Indian wrestlers who would swing huge solid wood clubs, strongman training has helped men develop incredibly strong, functional bodies that translate into real world application. It's also a gratifying practice; lifting a 60 kg log above your head for the first time is chest-thumpingly primal.

Sometimes lifting an object with a straight back (or neutral spine) is not possible, such as when picking up a couch. In strongman training, by learning to lift a stone, you're teaching your body to be strong in spinal flexion, which is the most common position people sustain a hernia of their vertebral disc. Had you trained your body to lift with your spine rounded, you may have prevented yourself from injuring your back while bending over to tie your shoes.

Calisthenics is rapidly gaining popularity in the world of movement as the rise of YouTube sensations make seemingly impossible feats of human performance look slightly less impossible. This type of strength training is very humbling, as it may take many years of disciplined practice before you are doing handstands or front levers (hanging from the bar with your arms outstretched and your body parallel to the floor).

Calisthenics holds the added benefit of requiring very minimal equipment, and the lack of extra weight allows your body to recover much easier from workouts. When holding an additional 100 kg on your back or in your hands, your central nervous system is depleted, which means calisthenics practitioners can train for longer and more frequently than powerlifters. If you haven't seen the physiques of calisthenics athletes, then search YouTube now. They are surely the most inspiring body shapes out of the training methods I have outlined here.

With any form of strength training, it should be mandatory that you seek professional coaching. You will save yourself years of wasted time, energy and most likely unnecessary injury with a few hundred dollars per month. I have had many brave men come to me with the confidence of 'years' of strength training, only to be reduced to a pile of sweaty goop after deadlifting sets of 50 kg.

"What about Crossfit?", You may ask. I have never personally coached Crossfit, but I have attended a few classes, and they ranged wildly from high-intensity interval training to strict Olympic lifting. If you can, find a club that demands minimal endurance training and focuses on the body as a holistic system. If your coach wants you to beat records every single workout, then that's probably not the right place for you to train as a busy man with a family and career. One thing that Crossfit does have is an incredible community, which - as we discussed in Chapter Four - can have incomparable benefits to your health. So feel free to mingle amongst your gym buddies and then tell your coach to shove it if he asks you to do another 5km run or ergo for the week.

That goes for the new craze of F45 too. The problem with these types of training is that they treat everyone the same. From amateur athletes, to new mums, to men working 70 hour weeks, everyone is treated equal, which in this case is wrong. Much like nutrition, exercise or movement practice is best treated individually. Everyone has different circumstances, different biomechanics and different internal biochemistry, each requiring different exercise programming.

One of the best ways to increase energy demand of the body is through movement complexity. As in the previous chapter, learning new complex movements is very challenging, and I have seen it work tremendously well for losing body fat. Parkour, dance, animal locomotion (not a train full of cats) and martial arts are all very progressive forms of 'exercise', and I highly encourage anyone interested to attend a class as soon as possible. In these disciplines, the movement patterns are rarely repeated too often. As opposed to running or cycling, where your body is moving in the same way over and over again, with a movement practice, you contort your muscles and joints in almost every way imaginable. You will not only enjoy learning a new skill, but you will also improve your body awareness and control, strength, mobility and body composition.

The reason we exchange cardio for strength training is again concerning cortisol management. Chronic cortisol elevation can destroy or guts, our immune system, our bone and muscle density and our brains. When we perform strength training, we do increase cortisol levels, but we also produce much higher levels of testosterone and growth hormone, which have been shown to increase muscle mass, reduce body fat and come with the myriad of other benefits that those hormones produce. Think about it this way, when you perform strength training for one hour, you are only exerting yourself for a maximum of twenty minutes, whereas if you go for a one hour run, you are exerting yourself for that full hour. For strength training, the benefits far outweigh the costs.

I have found calisthenics, or gymnastic strength training to be the best for becoming strong, lean and mobile without too much stress on your adrenal glands or your nervous system. As for yoga, I view this more as a spiritual practice that happens to include movement, so we'll discuss that in detail in the chapter entitled Ancient Wisdom.

My point in this chapter is not to insult or discourage you from cycling with your buddies every morning but to show you that there is a more efficient way to reach your physical goals, especially if those goals involve improving your body composition to the best of your ability. To throw my Dad under the bus again, he is a passionate cyclist and often complains about feeling smashed on the bike. His nervous system and adrenal glands are severely depleted. I tell him to eat more, but he doesn't believe me. Father knows best indeed.

Endurance training is better than nothing, but if you have the liberty of choosing which form of exercise you would like to do the next few decades, you might as well pick the one that's best for your body. Choose complex, non-repetitive movements that develop strength, mobility and coordination.

Chapter Sixteen

Becoming Mobile

"Those who do not move, do not notice their chains".

- *Rosa Luxemburg*

At the beginning of every client's journey, I ask them why are they seeking my help. There are about 15 common answers that range from getting better sleep, to improving their libido. The outcome that's usually third or fourth on their list is mobility.

Mobility is the degree to which you can control your body in end-range motion. Flexibility, on the other hand, is the amount of stretch that is available in a particular joint. An example of mobility is holding the splits with your feet elevated, think Jean-Claude Van Damme between two chairs in that wince-inducing scene in *Bloodsport*. Flexibility is laying on your back and pulling your leg toward you. Mobility is considered more appropriate for real world application, and is therefore the most desired of the two abilities.

As we have discussed in previous chapters, our environment is shaping us to be rather dysfunctional human beings. Our modern comforts have created a cast for our body to decay in. Our shoes, chairs, cars, phones, and laptops have bound us into a seated, hunched forward position.

We have a secret at 5EW. We promise individually tailored, personalised programs. That's right; no cookie-cutter Instagram on premises. However, if you were around long ...you would notice that most beginners have the same program. Why?

Well, because 99% of our members sit at a desk all day. Human beings are very similar to one another. We have genetic variances that cause slight differences, but the bulk of us respond to a physical stimulus in the same way. One of those ways is Wolff's law, that says the body will lay down more collagen to an area that bears the most weight. This means that when we do weight-bearing exercise, our bones become stronger. This also means that when you wear pointy-toed shoes, you develop bunions on your feet, and when you hang your neck forward to look at your phone, you force your vertebrae to lay down bone and mould to that deformed goose-neck position. Imagine the posture of our next generation.

So we respond to these modern casts in nearly identical ways:

1. A forward head and hyper-kyphotic (rounded) spine, due to tight pectoral muscles and neglected shoulder external rotators and retractors.
2. Weak abdominals and gluteal muscles.
3. Tight hip flexors and adductors.
4. Shortened Achilles tendons.

These deficiencies are what categorise 'executive posture syndrome'. Thankfully, we know how to fix it.

The solution is in new ways of movement, of course, but also with better nutrition. I've seen many cases of stubborn gym goers keep trying to regularly stretch, do yoga, etc., but they don't focus on holistic health. An underlying level of inflammation prevents them from making any serious improvements in a reasonable amount of time.

Mobility takes a long time to improve. Your cartilaginous structures in your joints regenerate over many, many months and so it's best not to delay mobility work. If you value mobility (if you've read this far, you should), it's important to start a practice as soon as you can. I began my journey with yoga. As I said in the opening section, this completely transformed how I felt within my body, and my whole family decided to join the yoga bandwagon with me. Several years later and I found gymnastics and movement culture.

Primarily, yogis achieve their level of mobility through lightness, spaciousness and breath, while gymnasts increase mobility through repetition and load. Take for example the Jefferson Curl. Imagine holding a weight in your hands while standing tall. Then curl your spine forward slowly, flexing vertebrae after vertebrae like a snail, until you are folding forward as far as you can and then reversing the undulation to reach the standing position. It's best to start this exercise with less than 10 kg in your hands and eventually - perhaps over several years - work your way to half your body weight. The added weight strengthens as well as lengthens the muscles and ligaments of the spine. This exercise can be performed daily for three sets of 10 reps. With the Jefferson Curl, you will be touching your toes in no time. That might sound like a trivial achievement, but it's life changing.

As modern, desk-bound humans, we've lost the ability to flex our spines; even worse is our inability to extend our spines. Imagine laying on your back, placing your heels to your buttocks and palms on the floor beside your ears. Now press up into a back bridge or wheel pose and straighten your elbows and knees. The vast majority of men aged 30 and above would struggle to lift off the floor. Our shoulders, upper back, abdominals and hip flexor muscles are so tight that any form of spinal extension may cause pain in the lower back, or even dizziness. This tightness is often accompanied with a shortened diaphragm and lung space, leading to breathing restrictions and ultimately less energy throughout your day.

This skill is harder to achieve without the help of a coach, but if you're willing; start standing with your back to a wall, about one foot away. Then, inhale to lift your spine, and begin to reach your palms over your head (fingers pointing to the floor) and backwards to the wall behind you. Over time your hands will get lower and lower toward the floor. Then you can start to practice with your feet elevated to knee height and then ultimately, you will be lying flat on the floor. There is likely no limit to the amount that you can practice this, in fact, the more often, the better for your spine and energy levels.

I am always amazed at how many human beings in the concrete jungle have lost some of their essential functions. To squat is to rest with the soles of your feet on the floor and your buttocks close to your heels. Billions of people in the developing world eat food, wait for the bus, talk amongst friends, and go to the toilet in a passive squat position. In a world where our spines have fused, our hips bound up and our ankles turned to solid rock, it makes it incredibly difficult for some people to get into this position for a even few seconds.

This inability to squat has a dysfunctional effect on your digestion, energy levels and sexual organs. Humans are very good at moving in and out of sitting on chairs, but the basic squatting movement has disappeared. As I mentioned before, but it bears repeating, the consequence of this is an epidemic of constipation. We have evolved to eliminate waste in a squatting position and so, when sitting down onto our ceramic thrones each morning, we strain and push until our blood vessels pop out of our eyes. This obviously isn't ideal.

For full and holistic health, this squatting position must become easy for you to rest in for at least 10 minutes. If you can't enter this position without falling backwards, hold onto something in front of you to keep your weight forward over your toes. The ultimate test is to hold a squat with your feet and knees together. This position deserves a lot of time. Be very patient.

Another foundation of human evolution is the passive hang. One of the biomechanical tests that we use is to time how long you can hold yourself hanging from a bar. Simply hold onto a bar overhead, lift your feet off the floor, relax and breathe. If you do not reach 2 minutes, you need to improve. If you do not reach 60 seconds, this is a concern. Frighteningly, one major predictor of all-cause mortality is grip strength relative to body weight[56] (another is how easily you can get up and down from the floor. Hint: don't use your hands). A short hang-time may be an indicator that you are carrying too much weight, that your forearm muscles are weak or even that you are overworked and undernourished. More sleep and food is a quick way to boost your grip strength and endurance, indicating a healthier, well-rested body.

This passive hang is unbelievably effective at decompressing the spine, releasing tight shoulders and naturally improving grip strength. If you have shoulder injuries or tightness in your upper back, spend five minutes hanging from a bar every day for 30 days and notice the profound change that occurs.

There's a reason that dancers of all kinds have incredible mobility. It's because they move their body in complex ways over and over again (if there is one key message from this chapter, it is repetition). Ido Portal brought the world something he calls *Movement Terminology*. This is a practice that develops our ability to articulate our spine in nonlinear patterns.

Your spine has roughly 50 joints that allow you to move in complex ways. Unfortunately, due to a sedentary lifestyle and lack of movement complexity, most of us have lost full control of our spine. Undulating your spine like a wave is seemingly impossible for most modern men. Being able to translate one vertebra on top of another (think egyptian dance) is also extremely difficult if untrained. But it can be done and should be practised enough that you gain maximum control over your spine.

This foundational practice has many benefits. Aside from the obvious fact that more range of motion is usually better than less, *Movement Terminology* prepares us for life. Life is nonlinear; it's unchoreographed and chaotic. If you're hit in a car accident with a neck of an 80-year-old, you're much more likely to sustain a serious injury than if you had the spine of a supple leopard (for this comparison, the leopard is licenced to drive a car). It may take years, but your spine can become supple. This is the part of you that connects your brain to the rest of your body. It must be cared for.

With these methods and accompanying nutrition, I have taken dozens of clients from chronic pain and poor mobility, to functional, mobile homo sapiens. If you practice these movements often enough, you will experience the same transformation of men gone before you. A mobile, pain-free body is essential for life satisfaction. It is hard to play with your kids and make love to your partner if your body doesn't respond the way you ask it. The first step to becoming mobile is to understand the importance of it. Then apply the techniques above. These are tried and true. Value them. Use them.

Chapter Seventeen

The Secret Weapon

"I am still learning".

- Michelangelo, age 87

The human body is adaptive. We provide it with a challenge, and it learns to overcome the challenge. Nowhere is this process more visible than in the realm of physical performance. The marvellous thing about physical performance is that it's increasingly linked to mental performance. The more confidently someone can control their body, the more they can control their mind. Thus, the secret weapon for a happy, functional life well into your senior years, is skill development.

Development of new skills is by far the best way to not only preserve the white matter of your brain, but to grow new nerve cells (neurogenesis) and also the connections between nerve cells (synaptogenesis)[57]. This process of overcoming challenges may have a dramatic impact on your long term brain health. From learning a language to balancing on a high wire, your brain must work overtime when developing a new skill. Preventing Alzheimer's and Parkinson's disease can actually be a whole lot of fun.

One of my most rewarding coaching experiences was helping a lovely lady through a particularly difficult part of her adult life. She was in her 50s and had struggled with a range of medical conditions from rheumatoid arthritis to severe anxiety. After a lifetime of bodily dissociation, she had nearly no control of her left arm. Take a moment to think how helpless she must have felt.

One morning, we began a session learning to throw one ball up in the air and catch it with the same hand. I gave her three balls to take home, and whenever she felt like it, she would practice throwing and catching the balls. I saw her every week, and we would spend 30 minutes learning to juggle, and 30 minutes practising breathwork and meditation. I watched her begin to lighten up, and in just two short months, she juggled three balls for a few seconds above her head. It was truly magical.

The best part wasn't that she could juggle, or even that she now felt that her left arm belonged to her. The best part of this experience was that she learnt that the mind and body are beautifully adaptable. She had (and now has) a deep sense of fulfilment from being able to do something she never thought she could. Many of our sessions were filled with laughter, smiles and pure joy at the wonder of learning a new skill.

I recognised that by taking this person out of her mind, and into her body, we were tapping into a different level of being. Science has suggested that learning to juggle increases the density of the corpus callosum of the brain[57], which is the portion that connects the left and right hemispheres. This increase in neuronal connection allows for faster thinking in critical situations. It's probably not the *Limitless* drug, but I'm sure that this attribute is highly sought after in your daily routine.

Another benefit of learning to juggle is that it forces you to be humble, and develop patience and persistence. It's interesting to watch how many people get frustrated at themselves for not knowing how to do something they have never practised before. Give someone three balls and tell them to start juggling, and they may have steam coming out of their ears in a few painful minutes. "Why are you so arrogant that you believe you can juggle without having ever done it before?", I ask. A lightbulb moment usually occurs in their heads. If it were easy, then everyone would be able to juggle, and it wouldn't be as special. Jimi Hendrix didn't just pick up a guitar and start playing it with his teeth. Appreciate the beauty in learning something new and your whole life will take a new form.

Next time an obstacle presents itself in your work environment, you can now view it as a fun challenge that you can learn from. Juggling, or any skill development for that matter, is a metaphor for learning in life. To paraphrase the great samurai warrior, Miyamoto Musashi, if you see the way in one thing, you will see it in everything.

Skill development can come in many forms. Balance is an often forgotten component in the fitness industry. How much can you honestly say that you perform movements - or to use the colloquial term, exercise - on one leg, or even on only your hands? It's unbelievable to think that the first step toward death for the majority of our elderly population is simply falling over. When we fall, we break a hip, get sent to a hospital, catch an illness and die. It seems to me then that the majority of focus in aged care facilities should be spent on developing balance.

Walking along a slackline (a tight bungee cord strung between two objects) has a tremendously positive effect on your brain. It forces you to focus in on a very specific task, a translatable skill that's surely in high demand in your professional arena. It forces your brain to send signals at the speed of light to your entire body. Invert right foot. Bend left knee. Lift right arm. Look up. All this happens in an unconscious flash. The stabilising muscles in your feet, knees and hips experience the most intense burning sensation you never thought possible. A strong lower body is essential for a functional life well into your senior years, as demonstrated by those thriving in *Blue Zone* destinations around the world.

When you have a child, you are forced to become a kid again. You spend more time on the floor than you have in decades, squatting, crawling and rolling around. If you haven't practised these movements in a while, you will have a difficult adjustment period. Your knees will hurt, your back will ache, and you will fall over your feet time and time again. Playing with my future children will be one of the highlights of my adult life, I'm sure of it. I know because I was lucky enough to have my Dad healthy and active when I was growing up. He remembers wrestling us three boys being some of the most joy-filled moments of fatherhood. I wish that same capacity for you.

In a recent interview, Ido Portal had said that happiness is not likely to be a good orientation for satisfaction in life. There is too much comfort and pleasure associated with happiness. Instead, orient yourself towards fearlessness. While you probably won't achieve a state of absolute fearlessness in this lifetime, you will learn to dance with fear. Whether it's learning a new language, to play hacky-sack, or to balance high up on a fence railing, there will be fear somewhere. Seek it out because where there is fear and discomfort, there is growth. As personal development guru Tony Robbins says, "If you're not growing, you're dying".

I encourage you to go out and learn something new. Choose a new skill that you have been putting off due to time commitments or otherwise. If possible, make it a movement-related skill and if you have them, involve your kids too. It could be a new sport, a martial art, yoga, rock climbing or circus. The more discomfort and fear behind it, the more change will occur and the happier you will become. Your kids will love you for taking on a new challenge, and your colleagues will envy your heightened levels of superhuman performance. Embrace fear. Enjoy life.

Chapter Eighteen

Ancient Wisdom

"Enlightenment is an accident, but some activities make you accident-prone".

- *Jiddu Krishnamurti*

In life, we have a few major turning points. For me, one of those was my motor-vehicle accident, where I was thrust into a world of health and wellness that I barely saw coming. The other was with the adoption of yoga.

Yogic practice began during the Vedic traditions in ancient India around 5,000 BCE. Then, it was mostly sitting, meditating and chanting, all to calm the fluctuations of the mind. Flash forward 7,000 years later, and the fluctuations of our mind are stronger than ever. As a society, we are plunging into a world of neuroticism, narcissism and materialism that is damaging the health and well-being of ourselves, our relationships, and the entire planet.

In this chapter, I want to outline the major benefits that a regular practice of yoga has on our mental and physical bodies. Although I haven't yet delved into the world of Tai Chi or QiGong, I have close relationships with people who practice these disciplines regularly and experience the same profound healing effects. When you look into the eyes of someone who knows the way, you acknowledge each other differently. The ancient wisdom of soft martial arts pours through them, and they understand the universe in a different, perhaps wholehearted way.

Cardiovascular disease is one of the largest causes of death in the Western world. We know, both from science and experience, that the cardiovascular system is closely linked with emotional stress. When we are stressed, our heart beats faster, or it might even palpitate, our face goes red, and blood pressure elevates. The most common time for a man to sustain a heart attack is between 6:00 a.m. and noon, when cortisol levels are at their peak. This one example illustrates the powerful link between the heart and emotions.

The practice of yoga, through stress reduction, has been shown to reduce the risk of cardiovascular disease[58]. As this illness is multifactorial, many parameters are usually measured, including cholesterol levels, blood pressure, heart rate, inflammation, and blood vessel damage.

To quote one study in particular:

"After one year, the yoga groups showed a significant reduction in number of anginal episodes per week, improved exercise capacity and a decrease in body weight. Serum total cholesterol, LDL cholesterol and triglyceride levels also showed greater reductions as compared with control group. Revascularization procedures were less frequently required in the yoga group. Coronary angiography repeated at one year showed that significantly more lesions regressed and fewer lesions progressed in the yoga group"[59].

Yoga and most of the practices found in this book have been shown to improve something called heart rate variability (HRV). Elite athletes and other peak-performers use HRV to measure their levels of recovery. It is the measurement of variation in the time interval between heartbeats. This provides critical information about the function of your autonomic system. Put simply, it measures how stressed your body is, and as we now understand, this has the biggest impact on your overall health above anything else. Yoga, along with nature walks and adequate sleep, increases HRV, which indicates a system that is relaxed and recovered, primed for performance[59].

To have such a profound effect on the largest cause of death in the West makes me believe this should be mandatory for companies to implement for their staff. The downstream effect on the economy from reduced healthcare costs, insurance, etc., is also worthy of further discussion. Those of you reading this who may be able to encourage your colleagues or employees to experience these effects should exercise that opportunity.

Our neurology is the least understood system of the human body. Every day we discover something new about how our brain and its chemicals work. Despite this, the research describing the benefits of yoga predominantly involve our nervous system. What's undeniable for any experienced practitioner of yoga, is the feeling we have after practice.

The effects of yoga on the neurological system are profound. From balancing neurotransmitters to increased levels of grey matter[60]. From changes in brain waves to permanent physical rewiring as a result of neuroplasticity, our brains are an incredible organ that allows us to feel the full spectrum of emotions, something unique to the human species.

Our major stress hormone cortisol directly destroys neurons in our hippocampus, which leads to a reduced ability to integrate short-term memory to long-term memory. When we meditate, we gain a much greater control of our HPA-axis, which governs cortisol secretion. This act of meditation undoubtedly leads to increased memory and concentration through the attenuation of the sympathetic nervous system.

Brain waves are the result of, and also control our state of being in the world. We have six activity levels of brain waves, measured in hertz (cycles per second):

1. Gamma 38-42hz.
2. Beta 12-38hz.
3. Alpha 8-12hz.
4. Theta 3-8hz.
5. Delta 0.5-3hz.
6. Infra-Low <0.5hz.

As Steven Cope suggests in his book *The Wisdom of Yoga*, brain waves can be altered through the practice of yoga.

"Brain wave activity begins to shift from the "beta waves" of regular wakefulness to somewhat longer, slower "alpha waves". We feel what it's like to inhabit a genuinely calm body. New research shows, too, that meditation produces identifiable changes in the brain. Meditation increases activity in areas of the brain associated with positive feelings, reduction in anxiety and faster recovery after negative provocation".

"We know that [meditation] promotes states of equanimity in several ways: The levels of stress hormones – epinephrine, norepinephrine, cortisol – are ratcheted down, calming the nervous system. Heart rate and blood pressure drop and the breathing rate slows as the body's need for oxygen is reduced. Metabolism slows. Muscle tension is relaxed significantly".

All of this is achieved through the activation of the parasympathetic nervous system. When we practice meditation, chanting and diaphragmatic breathing, we activate the vagus nerve, which is responsible for the 'rest and digest' functions of our body[61].

Yoga also affects our neurotransmitters. Through deep breathing, we can produce dopamine, which stimulates our reward centres of our brain[62]. However, the calming effects of yoga are also very noticeable. Part of this reason is the increase in production of GABA, a neurotransmitter that governs our feeling of calmness as well as our ability to sleep for eight hours unbroken throughout the night.

It's clear that yoga positively affects our neurophysiology, which as we will now see, results in greater feelings of happiness as we navigate this wonderful thing called life.

If we can make an abrupt, but serious segway; suicide is the largest cause of death in Australian men under the age of 50. This statistic is very disturbing for anyone who has gone through depression and knew what it means. Yoga played a significant role for me eliminating depression. The central area of our brain that governs fear and anxiety is the amygdala. It's been shown that meditation can reduce the activity and size of the amygdala after just a few weeks of practice[61].

One study involving depressed men of military service said:

"Subjects who participated in the yoga course demonstrated significant decreases in self-reported symptoms of depression and trait anxiety. Changes were also observed in acute mood, with subjects reporting decreased levels of negative mood and fatigue. Finally, there was a trend for higher morning cortisol levels compared to the control".

I can honestly say that yoga helped me through the trauma of my journey through early adulthood. This practice brought me closer to myself and opened me up to a new state of being. I was happier, calmer, and more self-assured with my decisions. This is mostly unexplainable on a personal level, but I am sure it was the result of this practice.

According to Dr Mario Martinez, author and longevity scientist, 75% of busy executives have gastrointestinal disorders. You don't need me to tell you that's a lot. What's the likely link? Stress.

Your central nervous system interacts with another nervous system located in your gut: the enteric nervous system. Yep, your gut pretty much has its own brain. You've experienced this connection before – those butterflies in your stomach are caused by an emotional response. To separate the mind and body would be ridiculous.

Cortisol affects the gut in many ways such as decreased nutrient absorption, plus an increased occurrence of bloating and constipation[63]. A chronic elevation of our primary stress hormone, cortisol, has been linked with many chronic gastrointestinal disorders. Crohn's disease, IBS, ulcerative colitis, and bowel cancers to name a few. Stress affects the gut in many ways, including disruption of bacteria and gut hormones, and increased intestinal permeability (leaky gut).

How then does yoga prevent this damage from occurring? By interrupting stress at the source. By affecting the neurochemistry, we affect the gut chemistry. This doesn't mean we can eat a whole pile of gluten, sugar, alcohol, and conventional dairy products and just throw in some yoga for gut health. With a healthy diet however, yoga can help alleviate many chronic digestive conditions. I know from experience, whenever I'm more stressed, my guts don't function as well.

If you're taking care of your nutrition, pay attention here. A simple yoga practice incorporating backbends, forward bends, twisting and side-bending, coupled with breathing and meditation could be the answer to your unhappy guts. One of my clients is a CEO of a large childhood trauma centre in Victoria. He regularly complained of gut distension and bloating from a few decades of less than perfect food choices. This man embarked on a 30 day yoga challenge and soon found a greater sense of mobility in his body and tranquillity in his belly. He continues to do yoga almost every day along with Adrienne and her 2.5 million YouTube subscribers.

I have uncovered much of the scientific benefits of yoga for almost the entire human body. From our brains to our belly, it's clear that a regular yoga practice has a profound effect on our physiology. I have experienced these effects in my own life, and I know many people around me who have had a tremendous boost in quality of life by including yoga in their weekly schedule. If you are in a position of responsibility and increased levels of stress, this practice may be the single most important lesson you take from this book. I encourage you to try 10 classes, whether they be in yoga, tai chi, qigong or any other soft martial art practice in your area. 10 classes allow you to experience different teachers and see the accumulative effects of the practice.

Om Shanti.

Part Four: Movement - Summary

Move intelligently and consciously, everyday.

1. Focus on a few movements you can do each day.
2. Examine how your environment dictates your movement patterns.
3. Purchase a Squatty Potty or Knees Up stool.

Incorporate strength training and movement complexity into your exercise schedule.

4. Lift heavy for optimal body composition and hormonal function.
    1. Calisthenics or gymnastics
    2. Strongman training or powerlifting
5. Explore new methods of movement.
    1. Surfing
    2. Rock-climbing
    3. Dance
    4. Martial Arts

Prioritise physical mobility as a necessity for life.

6. Make it your goal to touch your toes, do a back bridge or simply sit crossed-legged.

Learn something new and exciting.

7. Developing physical skills is essential to life.

Develop some ancient wisdom.

8. Practice ten yoga, qi-gong or tai chi classes, either online or in a studio.

Your Deserve It

"To live is the rarest thing in the world. Most people just exist".

- Oscar Wilde

Most of us are unaware of the degree of damage that having poor health has on the rest of our lives. We sacrifice so much of ourselves for career success, for our family, and for other people's ideals, that we forget who we are. Life can flash by in an instant, and all of a sudden you're 50 years old and have to spend the next five to 10 years trying to reclaim your youth.

The myriad of problems that come from poor health can be catastrophic. We start by getting out of shape, and we frequently become sick. We suffer from poor gut health and experience bloating, gas and constipation. We feel poorly within our bodies and experience back pain and stiffness in our neck. Our cognition begins to decline with mental fog, and we start to lose our memory. We have less desire for our partner, and we become sexually unattractive to them. Time and energy become our most precious resource as we fall into more stress, anxiety, and ultimately depression. We experience a lack of connection with ourselves and with others around us. Pleasures come and go, but in the end, deep down we are unhealthy, unhappy and unfulfilled.

The reasons for this regrettable existence are just as numerous. We work too much. We don't manage our stress levels with meditation, journaling, or walking in nature. Our sleep falls down our list of priorities, and we push on. We live in a polluted environment and clean ourselves and our homes with toxic products. We spend too much time on social media and watching television. We forget how to breathe properly. We eat unhealthy food and eat them on the run. We deprive our body of nutrients with quick-fix diets, and by starving ourselves. This forces us to rely on stimulants like sugar and caffeine instead of supplementing with vital minerals like zinc and magnesium. We drink alcohol to numb the pain or to lubricate our social inhibitions and be seen as 'fitting in'. We don't move enough, or in the right ways. We continually look for quick fixes as we desperately try to solve our problems.

But it's clear that these problems are more complicated, and require much more than just a magic pill or a one-trick pony. Instead, our health requires a holistic approach. We need to look at the human being in its entirety. While studying pre-medicine, we learnt about the biopsychosocial model of healthcare, that considers the social relationships and internal thoughts and emotions of the patient, as well as their physical health. Somewhere along the line, I feel like this model has been forgotten.

Throughout this book, you learned *The Four Pillars of Wellness*.

First, we focus on the mind. With techniques like meditation, journaling, breathwork, and belonging to a community, we can cut chronic stress off at the source and begin to appreciate and embrace life and ourselves more fully. With less stress or fear, and more happiness, our health immediately begins to transform.

Next, we discover the powerful effects that connecting back to nature has on our physiology. We begin to clean ourselves and our homes with healthy, plant-based, organic products. We supply our home with clean water and fresh air. We expose ourselves to the elements through heat and cold therapy. We dived into the science of sleep optimisation, and can now wake up well-rested every morning. We learnt that by doing something as basic as walking barefoot on the earth, we develop a connection with the planet to instantly reduce the hyperactivity of our nervous system.

Then we explored nutrition, and the complexities that are associated with this emotionally charged topic. Remember that one man's fuel is another man's poison, and many benefits of this section must be achieved only through trial and error. We know what foods to avoid to reduce inflammation and improve our health span. We understand that starving ourselves is not the answer, but instead we should feed the body nutrients that it wants and needs. Supplementation is now simplified, and you can rest easy knowing you no longer have to buy exotic herbs that are blessed by Nepalese monks on the top of a sacred mountain.

Finally, we shifted our thinking around what it means to move. You now no longer partake in exercise but a movement practice. You understand that this practice occurs all day and night. Strength is now a priority for you as you now know the hormonal benefits and primal thrill that comes with this practice. You understand the importance of mobility, and integrating the development of new skills into your life. Lastly, you are fascinated by the ancient traditions of yoga, tai chi, and qigong, and the longevity boosting qualities that these movement practices have. You move because you're human and you enjoy it.

Your health, and equally as importantly, your happiness is a product of the four pillars above. It's imperative that you identify which areas need the most improvement and start implementing the lessons in each of the chapters within.

However, I understand that there is enough content in this book to fill an entire day, and not leave any room for the other activities that fill your life. Integrate the lessons that will bring you the most bang for your time-based buck, and if possible, couple those activities with some other daily routine. For example, perhaps you can now meditate, or journal on your commute to work or in an infrared sauna. Maybe you can couple your movement practice with being outside, barefoot amongst nature. Whichever the method you choose, don't allow yourself to become overwhelmed.

But of course, you are probably looking for the cheat notes; the top actions for an outstanding body and mind. If overwhelm is sounding familiar, I recommend starting with the following:

1.   Learn to breathe efficiently
2.   Optimise your sleep
3.   Complete the *Fresh Start*
4.   Move in new and complex ways for at least four hours each week.

My health journey has taken years of research as well as trial and error to get to this point. With this book, I merely want you to grasp the major concepts of what I have put forward. I want you to know that health does not need to be complicated, it does not need to be expensive, and it certainly does not need to be restrictive.

However, the most important lesson is that I want you to know that you deserve outstanding health. You deserve to live a long, healthy, vibrant and active life. You deserve to play with your great grandchildren and to enjoy a full and rich life, right up until you pass. Those closest and most dear to you are counting on you. It's time to show them how full of life you really are.

Appendix One

Where to Next?

If you're seeking the transformations that the dedicated men in this book have achieved, then all you need to do is follow the same path. By focusing on the mind, exposure to nature, maintaining proper nutrition and practising healthy movement, you are capable of reshaping your health and becoming the ultimate boss, lover, and father. You'll begin to have more energy, improve your tolerance to stress, and as the king of all bonuses, also look and feel good naked.

Jordan codeveloped the world's most comprehensive 12 week program that takes you through this holistic process. In just 84 days, you can completely transform how you look and feel on the inside and out.

Visit www.theultimatereboot.com for more details.

To find more on Jordan, visit www.jordantravers.com. Here you can continue your education, browse Jordan's events schedule, and subscribe to his newsletter.

And of course, if you enjoyed this book, you are welcome to leave a review on Amazon.

Appendix Two

What Does Success Look Like?

Nick Bletsas is one of my longest-standing clients who started with me in early 2015. He always struggled to maintain a consistent movement practice as he would quickly become burnt out and fall sick. Over time I have had the privilege to watch this now 32-year-old man become a true athlete. In two years he has transformed his body by losing nearly 9 kg of fat and adding another 9.5 kg of lean muscle. With the methods that he has applied in this book from the *Fresh Start* to community ice baths, Nick now sits at a lean 6% body fat all year, while running his graphic design and signage business out of Melbourne. His strength is unbelievable for someone who trains a few times per week, being able to squat with 120 kg on his back at 70 kg bodyweight. By eating more food than he ever has, Nick now has unlimited energy, is stronger than ever and hasn't been sick in over a year.

"My journey into movement, mindset, and myself began with coach Jordan in 2015, when I returned to training after a three-year hiatus due to over-training. Coach Jordan quickly gave me the tools to change my mindset towards training – helping me listen to my body, increase my training capacity and obtain tangible results through the wealth of knowledge that he shared with me on nutrition, meditation, movement, mobility, and life. I came back to training without a clear idea of what I wanted to achieve, and after being guided by Jordan for a short time, it became clear that I was in skillful hands. I quickly found my passion for movement and strength training again, and Jordan's guidance gave me the skills to set realistic goals. and work towards them progressively. With this new insight, I was able to go above and beyond anything I had ever achieved before in my training and has helped set a new benchmark for myself. Jordan is always enthusiastic towards coaching, and his willingness to share his abundant knowledge makes me feel very proud to have him in my corner. My journey with Jordan has given me an incredible new skill set and access to a better me. Jordan is a fantastic coach, human, and friend, and if you have the opportunity to have him in your corner expect amazing things!".

- Nicholas Bletsas, Director at Gramata Design Studio

As a coach, you get to meet some incredible people throughout your career. One of those men is Mr Andrew Hollo. Andrew was healthy for his entire young-adult life, but something happened when he turned 40. He began to put on body fat, develop back pain, and was feeling weak within his body. With a baby boy now growing up, Andrew had to act to be the father he knew his boy deserved. As a super-busy, independent consultant, Andrew used to struggle with healthy food choices on the run. He would take whatever he could get at meetings, conferences, and workshops which left him with a caffeine addiction and an oversized belly. Over time, Andrew has gradually adopted healthy lifestyle changes from the use of cold showers and infrared saunas, to prioritising movement and healthy nutrition. Over the three years that I have known Andrew, he values his health more than ever, and is seeing the benefits reaped across all areas of life.

"I was a super-stressed, caffeine-addicted, sugar-dependent, under-slept self-employed, 50-year-old business owner, husband, and father of a small boy. Jordan has provided me with a vision of what my better self can be, coaching on how to get there, encouragement when I fail, and even more encouragement when I don't fail. Now, two years later, I'm a productively-stressed, well-slept, healthy eating, self-employed business owner, husband, and father. In that time, my income has risen, my wife loves my new body, and I can wrestle my now 8-year-old boy all afternoon".

- Andrew Hollo, Director at Workwell Consulting

Gregory Nicolau is a clinical psychologist, CEO, and serial entrepreneur, having a hugely positive impact on childhood trauma treatment in Australia. He started out in the military, where he learnt to climb rope, perform one arm pushups, and analyse the psychology of his seniors. At 55 years old, Gregory arrived to me with the intention of having fun, and remaining as youthful as possible. Chronic stress throughout his career left him with an oversized belly and terrible gut health. He complained of sore, tight muscles and joints, and often lacked the energy to complete his workouts. Gregory now practices yoga nearly every day, has completed multiple *Fresh Starts* and diligently uses supplements to keep his digestion functioning optimally. He can now manage his stress levels at work, is the most mobile he's been in decades, and has enough energy to finish his workouts and even terrorise me afterwards.

"They say that the only problem with youth is that it is wasted on the young. Jordan is a young man going places, and he is definitely not wasting his youth. He has been my coach for two years, and in that time, I have found him to be very considered in his approach to our work together. He manages to persevere with my inconsistent approach to his instructions, and my mischief (think grumpy old man) is dealt with in his calm and steady manner. He is incredibly knowledgeable about all things relating to the mechanics and 'organics' of the body. He is extraordinarily impressive for one so young!".

- Gregory Nicolau, Founder / CEO at Australian Childhood Trauma Group.

It's not easy to undergo a health transformation after relocating half way across the globe but Englishman, Greg Braun decided to do exactly that. Soon after arriving in Melbourne, Greg started training with me and completed the *Fresh Start* along with some basic strength training. Along with his new perspective on nutrition, he began taking zinc and magnesium supplements regularly. In just his first seven months, Greg added 5.2kg of muscle to his frame and lost 6.2% body fat, which is a significant transformation of his physique. We also had some fun exploring the Wim Hof Method breathing technique and zero degree Community Ice Baths. From a modest 12kg kettlebell, we have now worked up to multiple repetitions of 130+kg deadlift, suggesting that Greg's strength has increased out of sight. There's no doubt that Greg's newfound passion for health and fitness is paying dividends to all other areas of his life.

"I was lucky enough to land Jordan as my PT upon joining my very first ever gym. And boy does he know his shit. Jordan's applied areas of expertise is extensive and his passion, relentless. He has been a significant part of my (well needed) journey to find better balance and make more educated choices when it comes to health, fitness and wellbeing. His unwavering attention to technique is his strength and while his makes for a tougher training session, I feel has taken me further, quicker. There is much about our sessions together that will stay with me – but above all it is how he makes simplifying the complex and makes learning fun. Everyone needs a Jordan in their life!"

- Greg Braun, REA Group

As an anaesthetist at both public and private hospitals, Chief Medical Officer for motor racing in Australia, and an emergency helicopter retrieval physician, Brent May knows a lot about the human body. But he had sacrificed his health for the health of others for nearly two decades. Throughout a busy day in theatre, he would consume excessive caffeine and sugar to get him through. He was taking prescription medication for chronic pain and indigestion, and he had become more out of shape than he was used to. After completing just the *Fresh Start*, Brent was able to come off his medication. It took a lot of work to uncover his biomechanical imbalances and fix them, but after almost two years of personal training, yoga and physical therapy, Brent is now pain-free. Although he doesn't admit that it's a priority, Brent has had fantastic body composition results too. In his first ten months, he dropped 6.4% body fat and added 6.7 kg of lean muscle to his frame. He now understands his body better than ever by focusing on eating significantly more healthy food to keep him going through an intense work schedule. He also makes use of an infra-red sauna and prioritises daily movement as a major part of his life.

"After several years of poor lifestyle habits including diet, alcohol and a stressful lifestyle, Jordan really helped change my life with his enthusiasm and knowledge. His focus on what really works and the evidence behind it really helped me become healthier, leaner and most importantly, happy and pain free. His holistic approach including movement, alignment, strength and diet has made a real difference to my life. Thanks Jordan."

- Brent May, Specialist anaesthetist and pre-hospital care physician. MBBS, FANZCA, MSc (Trauma)

I have peppered the story of Vince Burzomi sporadically throughout this book, and that's because he is truly inspiring. Weighing 199 kg, it was no easy feat for him to walk into a holistic health centre in a town that's known for its green smoothies and yoga studios. At 40 years old, a lifetime of ill-informed diet choices led Vince to become dangerously overweight and incredibly unhappy. Running one of the busiest mechanic shops in Melbourne, he survived off ten cappuccino's each day. He was always sick and suffered from chronic back pain, painful digestion and oppressive lethargy. His one wish was to walk across the road to watch his boys play football, but with insulin levels through the roof, Vince was diabetic and needed help. Through interventions in nutrition, lifestyle, movement, and mindset, Vince is now on top of the world. In two years, Vince is now swimming in his old shirts, he has put on a stack of muscle and is the strongest he has ever been in his entire life. His blood markers have improved out of sight to now become medically healthy. He no longer gets back pain, is never sick and has enough energy to walk across the city and dance with his youngest son all night long.

And that's what it's all about.

References

1. 4102.0 - Australian Social Trends. (2010, June). Retrieved Oct 23, 2017, from http://www.abs.gov.au/AUSSTATS/abs@.nsf/Lookup/4102.0Main+Features30Jun+2010

2. Biddulph, S. (2010). The new manhood: The handbook for a new kind of man. Finch Publishing.

3. Sansone, R. A., & Sansone, L. A. (2010). Gratitude and well being: The benefits of appreciation. Psychiatry (Edgmont), 7(11), 18.

4. Good, D. J., Lyddy, C. J., Glomb, T. M., Bono, J. E., Brown, K. W., Duffy, M. K., ... & Lazar, S. W. (2016). Contemplating mindfulness at work: an integrative review. Journal of Management, 42(1), 114-142.

5. Lutz, A., Brefczynski-Lewis, J., Johnstone, T., & Davidson, R. J. (2008). Regulation of the neural circuitry of emotion by compassion meditation: effects of meditative expertise. PloS one, 3(3), e1897.

6. Kox, M., van Eijk, L. T., Zwaag, J., van den Wildenberg, J., Sweep, F. C., van der Hoeven, J. G., & Pickkers, P. (2014). Voluntary activation of the sympathetic nervous system and attenuation of the innate immune response in humans. Proceedings of the National Academy of Sciences, 111(20), 7379-7384.

7. Why Is Nose Breathing Important for Optimal Health and Fitness?. (2016, July 30). Retrieved October 12, 2017, from https://articles.mercola.com/sites/articles/archive/2016/07/30/buteyko-breathing.aspx

8. Indoor Air Quality (IAQ). (2017, September 1). Retrieved October 12, 2017, from https://www.epa.gov/indoor-air-quality-iaq

9. How Toxic Is Your Home? - Griffith University. (n.d.). Retrieved October 12, 2017, from https://www.griffith.edu. au/environment-planning-architecture/ecocentre/news-events/articles/how-toxic-is-your-home

10. Levine, H., Jørgensen, N., Martino-Andrade, A., Mendiola, J., Weksler-Derri, D., Mindlis, I., ... & Swan, S. H. (2017). Temporal trends in sperm count: a systematic review and meta-regression analysis. Human Reproduction Update, 1-14.

11. Bohn, S., & Bircher, A. J. (2001). Phenoxyethanol-induced urticaria. Allergy, 56(9), 922-923.

12. Sher, L. (2013). Low testosterone levels may be associated with suicidal behavior in older men while high testosterone levels may be related to suicidal behavior in adolescents and young adults: a hypothesis. International journal of adolescent medicine and health, 25(3), 263-268.

13. Research | Protect Your Family from EMF Pollution - EMF Analysis. (n.d.). Retrieved October 12, 2017, from https://www.emfanalysis.com/research/

14. Wyde, M., Cesta, M., Blystone, C., Elmore, S., Foster, P., Hooth, M., ... & Walker, N. (2016). Report of Partial findings from the National Toxicology Program Carcinogenesis Studies of Cell Phone Radiofrequency Radiation in Hsd: Sprague Dawley® SD rats (Whole Body Exposure). bioRxiv, 055699.

15. Bortkiewicz, A., Gadzicka, E., & Szymczak, W. (2017). Mobile phone use and risk for intracranial tumors and salivary gland tumors-A meta-analysis. International journal of occupational medicine and environmental health.

16. Ferriss, T. (2010). The 4-hour body: An uncommon guide to rapid fat-loss, incredible sex, and becoming superhuman. Harmony.

17. Johnson, J. (n.d.) Research. Retrieved from https://www.emfanalysis.com/research/

18. Research news - Office plants boost well-being ... - University of Exeter. (2013, July 9). Retrieved October 12, 2017, from http://www.exeter.ac.uk/news/research/title_306119_en.html

19. Chasset, F., Soria, A., Moguelet, P., Mathian, A., Auger, Y., Francès, C., & Barete, S. (2016). Contact dermatitis due to ultrasound gel: A case report and published work review. The Journal of dermatology, 43(3), 318-320.

20. Ali, B., Al-Wabel, N. A., Shams, S., Ahamad, A., Khan, S. A., & Anwar, F. (2015). Essential oils used in aromatherapy: A systemic review. Asian Pacific Journal of Tropical Biomedicine, 5(8), 601-611.

21. The regulation of menstrual cycle and its relationship to the ... - NCBI. (n.d.). Retrieved October 12, 2017, from https://www.ncbi.nlm.nih.gov/pubmed/3716780

22. Xu, C., Zhang, J., Mihai, D. M., & Washington, I. (2014). Light-harvesting chlorophyll pigments enable mammalian mitochondria to capture photonic energy and produce ATP. J Cell Sci, 127(2), 388-399.

23. Kihara, T., Miyata, M., Fukudome, T., Ikeda, Y., Shinsato, T., Kubozono, T., ... & Lee, S. (2009). Waon therapy improves the prognosis of patients with chronic heart failure. Journal of cardiology, 53(2), 214-218.

24. Vatansever, F., & Hamblin, M. R. (2012). Far infrared radiation (FIR): its biological effects and medical applications. Photonics & lasers in medicine, 1(4), 255-266.

25. Ferriss T. (2014, April 10). Are Saunas the Next Big Performance-Enhancing "Drug"? | The Blog .... Retrieved October 12, 2017, from https://tim.blog/2014/04/10/saunas-hyperthermic-conditioning-2/

26. Patrick, R.P. (2016, February 15). Cold Shocking the Body - FoundMyFitness. Retrieved October 12, 2017, from https://www.foundmyfitness.com/reports/cold-stress.pdf

27. Vosselman, M. J., Vijgen, G. H., Kingma, B. R., Brans, B., & van Marken Lichtenbelt, W. D. (2014). Frequent extreme cold exposure and brown fat and cold-induced thermogenesis: a study in a monozygotic twin. PloS one, 9(7), e101653.

28. Tsunetsugu, Y., Park, B. J., & Miyazaki, Y. (2010). Trends in research related to "Shinrin-yoku"(taking in the forest atmosphere or forest bathing) in Japan. Environmental health and preventive medicine, 15(1), 27.

29. Park, B. J., Tsunetsugu, Y., Kasetani, T., Kagawa, T., & Miyazaki, Y. (2010). The physiological effects of Shinrin-yoku (taking in the forest atmosphere or forest bathing): evidence from field experiments in 24 forests across Japan. Environmental health and preventive medicine, 15(1), 18.

30. Morita, E., Fukuda, S., Nagano, J., Hamajima, N., Yamamoto, H., Iwai, Y., ... & Shirakawa, T. (2007). Psychological effects of forest environments on healthy adults: Shinrin-yoku (forest-air bathing, walking) as a possible method of stress reduction. Public health, 121(1), 54-63.

31. Bowman, K., & Lewis, J. (2014). Move Your DNA: Restore Your Health Through Natural Movement. Propriometrics Press.

32. Bratman, G. N., Hamilton, J. P., Hahn, K. S., Daily, G. C., & Gross, J. J. (2015). Nature experience reduces rumination and subgenual prefrontal cortex activation. Proceedings of the national academy of sciences, 112(28), 8567-8572.

33. Qureshi, I. A., & Mehler, M. F. (2014). Epigenetics of sleep and chronobiology. Current neurology and neuroscience reports, 14(3), 432.

34. Cappuccio, F. P., D'Elia, L., Strazzullo, P., & Miller, M. A. (2010). Sleep duration and all-cause mortality: a systematic review and meta-analysis of prospective studies. Sleep, 33(5), 585-592.

35. Goh, V. H. H., & Tong, T. Y. Y. (2010). Sleep, sex steroid hormones, sexual activities, and aging in Asian men. Journal of andrology, 31(2), 131-137.

36. Lack, L. C., Gradisar, M., Van Someren, E. J., Wright, H. R., & Lushington, K. (2008). The relationship between insomnia and body temperatures. Sleep medicine reviews, 12(4), 307-317.

37. Price, W. A., & Nguyen, T. (2016). Nutrition and physical degeneration: a comparison of primitive and modern diets and their effects. EnCognitive.com.

38. Shanahan, C. (2017). Deep nutrition: Why your genes need traditional food. Flatiron Books.

39. Keith, L. (2009). The vegetarian myth: food, justice, and sustainability. PM Press.

40. Arnold, L. E., Lofthouse, N., & Hurt, E. (2012). Artificial food colors and attention-deficit/hyperactivity symptoms: conclusions to dye for. Neurotherapeutics, 9(3), 599-609.

41. Visser, J., Rozing, J., Sapone, A., Lammers, K., & Fasano, A. (2009). Tight junctions, intestinal permeability, and autoimmunity. Annals of the New York Academy of Sciences, 1165(1), 195-205.

42. Rehm, J., Baliunas, D., Borges, G. L., Graham, K., Irving, H., Kehoe, T., ... & Roerecke, M. (2010). The relation between different dimensions of alcohol consumption and burden of disease: an overview. Addiction, 105(5), 817-843.

43. Vartanian, L. R., Schwartz, M. B., & Brownell, K. D. (2011). Effects of soft drink consumption on nutrition and health: a systematic review and meta-analysis. American journal of public health.

44. Schaefer, E. J., Gleason, J. A., & Dansinger, M. L. (2009). Dietary fructose and glucose differentially affect lipid and glucose homeostasis. The Journal of nutrition, 139(6), 1257S-1262S.

45. Takeaway coffee cups piling up in landfill as Australia's caffeine habit soars. Whyte, S. (2016). Retrieved from http://www.abc.net.au/news/2016-02-03/takeaway-coffee-cups-piling-up-in-landfill/7136926

46. Gilden, R. C., Huffling, K., & Sattler, B. (2010). Pesticides and health risks. Journal of Obstetric, Gynecologic, & Neonatal Nursing, 39(1), 103-110.

47. Khan, N., & Mukhtar, H. (2013). Tea and health: studies in humans. Current pharmaceutical design, 19(34), 6141-6147.

48. Sikorski, A. (2017). 2014 NICE cholesterol guidelines. Br J Gen Pract, 67(663), 446-446.

49. Mahler, M. (n.d.). Testosterone Is Great but Is Dihydrotestosterone the King of All Male .... Retrieved October 13, 2017, from http://mikemahler.com/articles-videos/hormone-optimization/testosterone-is-great-but-is-dihydrotestosterone-the-king-of-all-male-androgens

50. Jahnen-Dechent, W., & Ketteler, M. (2012). Magnesium basics. Clinical kidney journal, 5(Suppl_1), i3-i14.

51. Fasano, A. (2012). Zonulin, regulation of tight junctions, and autoimmune diseases. Annals of the New York Academy of Sciences, 1258(1), 25-33.

52. Campbell-McBride, N. (2010). Gut and psychology syndrome: natural treatment for autism, ADD/ADHD, dyslexia, dyspraxia, depression. Schizophrenia.

53. Perlmutter, D. (2015). Brain Maker: The Power of Gut Microbes to Heal and Protect Your Brain-for Life. Hachette UK.

54. Feingold, B. F. (1975). Hyperkinesis and learning disabilities linked to artificial food flavors and colors. AJN The American Journal of Nursing, 75(5), 797-803.

55. Evans, P. (n.d.). Kids food. Retrieved from https://thepaleoway.com/blog/kids-food/

56. Sayer, A. A., & Kirkwood, T. B. (2015). Grip strength and mortality: a biomarker of ageing?. Lancet (London, England), 386(9990), 226.

57. Scholz, J., Klein, M. C., Behrens, T. E., & Johansen-Berg, H. (2009). Training induces changes in white-matter architecture. Nature neuroscience, 12(11), 1370-1371.

58. Manchanda, S. C., Narang, R., Reddy, K. S., Sachdeva, U., Prabhakaran, D., Dharmanand, S., ... & Bijlani, R. (2000). Retardation of coronary atherosclerosis with yoga lifestyle intervention. The Journal of the Association of Physicians of India, 48(7), 687-694.

59. Vinay, A. V., Venkatesh, D., & Ambarish, V. (2016). Impact of short-term practice of yoga on heart rate variability. International journal of yoga, 9(1), 62.

60. Cope, S. (2006). The wisdom of yoga: A seeker's guide to extraordinary living. Bantam.

61. The Science behind Yoga (n.d.). Retrieved from http://www.artofliving.org/yoga/yoga-for-beginners/science-behind-yoga

62. Woolery, A., Myers, H., Sternlieb, B., & Zeltzer, L. (2004). A yoga intervention for young adults with elevated symptoms of depression. Alternative therapies in health and medicine, 10(2), 60.

63. Martinez, M. (2014). The MindBody Code: How to Change the Beliefs that Limit Your Health, Longevity, and Success. Sounds True.

About Jordan Travers

Jordan Travers is a personal trainer and holistic health coach based in Melbourne Australia. He specialises in personal transformation for high performance individuals who want to increase their productivity and life-satisfaction through the optimisation of health.

When he was 16, Jordan crashed a moped at 60 miles and hour, breaking bones and crushing his trachea, which placed him in a coma. The journey through intense medical and rehabilitative procedures was completely life changing and propelled him into health and wellness.

Jordan has consciously turned away from practitioner models of health, and has instead opted to transform men's lives by becoming one of the most highly regarded and influential staff at Australia's top holistic gym. He has personally coached over 100 clients one on one, and has influenced several hundred more in group settings. Many of his clients are successful business owners and executives, who sacrifice their health for their career, and seek Jordan's help to reclaim their vitality.

In his spare time, Jordan lectures and runs education programmes for coaches and gym owners on how to get better results with their clients, as well as with their own training. He also hosts personal transformation retreats for his clients in beautiful destinations around the world.

www.jordantravers.com